Maths Learning
Difficulties, Dyslexia and Dyscalculia
Second Edition

Steve Chinn

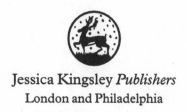

Jessica Kingsley *Publishers*
London and Philadelphia

Table 4.1 is reproduced from Chinn, S.J. and Ashcroft, J.R. (2017) *Mathematics for Dyslexics and Dyscalculics: A Teaching Handbook.* 4th edn. Chichester: Wiley with kind permission from Wiley. The first part of Chapter 22 is reproduced from Chinn, S.J. (2012) 'The Power of Estimation.' *Special (nasen)*, March 2012 with kind permission from nasen.

First published in 2019
by Jessica Kingsley Publishers
73 Collier Street
London N1 9BE, UK
and
400 Market Street, Suite 400
Philadelphia, PA 19106, USA

www.jkp.com

Library of Congress Cataloging in Publication Data
A CIP catalog record for this book is available from the Library of Congress

British Library Cataloguing in Publication Data
A CIP catalogue record for this book is available from the British Library

ISBN 978 1 78592 579 5
eISBN 978 1 78450 989 7

Printed and bound in Great Britain

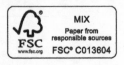

Maths Learning Difficulties, Dyslexia and Dyscalculia

by the same author

Addressing the Unproductive Classroom Behaviours of Students with Special Needs
ISBN 978 1 84905 050 0
eISBN 978 0 85700 357 7

of related interest

Understanding Dyscalculia and Numeracy Difficulties
A Guide for Parents, Teachers and Other Professionals
Patricia Babtie and Jane Emerson
ISBN 978 1 84905 390 7
eISBN 978 0 85700 754 4

Specific Learning Difficulties – What Teachers Need to Know
Diana Hudson
Illustrated by Jon English
ISBN 978 1 84905 590 1
eISBN 978 1 78450 046 7

The Parents' Guide to Specific Learning Difficulties
Information, Advice and Practical Tips
Veronica Bidwell
ISBN 978 1 78592 040 0
eISBN 978 1 78450 308 6

101 Inclusive and SEN Maths Lessons
Fun Activities and Lesson Plans for Children Aged 3–11
Claire Brewer and Kate Bradley
ISBN 978 1 78592 101 8
eISBN 978 1 78450 364 2
Part of the 101 Inclusive and SEN Lessons *series*

Dyslexia is My Superpower (Most of the Time)
Margaret Rooke
Forewords by Professor Catherine Drennan and Loyle Carner
ISBN 978 1 78592 299 2
eISBN 978 1 78450 606 3

The Illustrated Guide to Dyslexia and Its Amazing People
Kate Power and Kathy Iwanczak Forsyth
Foreword by Richard Rogers
ISBN 978 1 78592 330 2
eISBN 978 1 78450 647 6 3

Contents

Introduction

After 14 years of teaching in mainstream schools, in 1981 I took up a post which would make me the first Head of a new specialist secondary school for dyslexic boys. As a science teacher I was given the job of teaching mathematics to twelve very dyslexic students. I had been a very successful teacher in mainstream, but I was about to find out that I did not have the skills to teach my new students effectively.

In that brief biographical paragraph is the raison d'être for the next 30 years or so of my professional life and one person's realisation that specialist teacher training is essential if children who experience specific learning difficulties in maths are to be educated to the same standards of achievement as their peers.

Back in the 1980s very little was known about dyslexia's impact on learning maths and certainly we did not use the word 'dyscalculia'.

In 2019 mathematics learning difficulties and dyscalculia remain behind dyslexia in terms of research and understanding, but current knowledge is getting stronger and more research is being published. The rise of neuropsychology and brain scans is pushing our knowledge forward. However, this book is rooted in the classroom and thus about the pragmatics of teaching and learning.

One of my dreams is to see similar levels of acceptance and understanding in education for dyscalculia and maths learning difficulties (LD). The second goal is the training of a body of assessors, specialist teachers and learning support assistants. The third goal is that there will be a much greater recognition and acceptance of an adjusted pedagogy for maths learning difficulties led by our Government.

This short book can only give an overview of the many issues that are involved in mathematics learning difficulties and dyscalculia, but it is an overview that should highlight problems and point towards understanding and interventions. There are some themes that run through the book, for example, using key facts in a developmental way. The themes acknowledge the need to constantly revisit topics and extend them, building on secure foundations.

A pragmatic mantra: take the intervention back to the beginning and then proceed at a pace and with a style to match the needs of the student.

At the end of the book there is a list of References and Further Reading, some written by me, for those who wish to follow up any particular aspects or topics in more detail. My video tutorials, Maths Explained, show in detail how I teach maths.

Chapter 1

Dyslexia, Dyscalculia and Maths Learning Difficulties

As our knowledge of the theoretical bases of learning difficulties has improved so has awareness in schools. It would be beneficial to include that knowledge in all teacher training, coupled with pragmatic intervention methods, so that it is available at that critical interface between learner and teacher. There is a long way to go, but we have started.

The concept of comorbidity or co-occurrence of learning difficulties and their influences is now recognised. I was unaware in 1981 that my students, who were identified as dyslexic, could also have very significant difficulties with maths. This was not a unique situation at that time. We in the UK teaching profession were unaware of Asperger syndrome. We didn't understand attention deficit hyperactivity disorder (ADHD) or dyspraxia. Although Kosc had written about dyscalculia in 1974 only a few teachers were aware of its existence, but they were certainly well aware of underachievement in maths. Not many years ago people argued, often quite vehemently, as to whether dyslexia was 'dyslexia' or 'specific learning difficulty' or even 'specific learning difficulties/ dyslexia' and that's before we get to the discussions on 'difficulty' and 'disability'. These arguments did not include anything about the influence of dyslexia and other learning difficulties on learning maths.

There was a long definition of 'learning disabilities', the then alternative term used for dyslexia in the USA (Kavanagh and Truss

1988, p.550). As you read it, note how comprehensive it is regarding the influences, factors and co-occurring issues involved in LD:

> Learning disabilities is a generic term that refers to a heterogeneous group of disorders manifested by significant difficulties in the acquisition of listening, speaking, reading, writing, reasoning or mathematical abilities or of social skills. These disorders are intrinsic to the individual and presumed to be due to central nervous system dysfunction. Even though a learning disability may occur concomitantly with other handicapping conditions (e.g., sensory impairment, mental retardation, social and emotional disturbance), with socio-environmental influences (e.g., cultural differences, insufficient or inappropriate instruction, psychogenic factors) and especially with attention deficit disorder, all of which may cause learning problems, a learning disability is not the direct result of those conditions or influences.

Let me pick out the word 'heterogeneous'. Recent research on dyscalculia has described it as a heterogeneous condition, that is, there is not one single profile. We have to look at a range of potentially contributing factors (see Chapter 2).

The pioneering work of Sharma in the USA on maths difficulties was not known at that time in the UK, nor his journals, *Focus on Learning Problems in Mathematics* and *Math Notebook*. He remains a leading pragmatist in the field.

After an initial flurry of interest from the Department of Education in the UK around the millennium, interest in dyscalculia seems to have waned somewhat. The definition below is the one that the Department for Education and Skills published back in 2001. It has not been refreshed.

> Dyscalculia is a condition that affects the ability to acquire mathematical skills. Dyscalculic learners may have difficulty understanding simple number concepts, lack an intuitive grasp of numbers and

have problems learning number facts and procedures. Even if they produce a correct answer, or use a correct method, they may do so mechanically and without confidence. (DfES 2001, p.2)

Even though this definition is somewhat succinct, it is informative. My understandings of the various features covered in the definition are as follows:

It states that these learners have problems with numbers and thus the quantities represented by the (many) symbols used in maths. This infers problems at the very early stages of maths and thus, for children, the first maths experiences they meet. The use of the word 'intuitive' suggests an inborn ability to deal with numbers/quantities. This should not preclude successful intervention for learners who need to develop that facility later in childhood. We need to remember that there is often a big difference between what children can repeat or chant and what they understand and thus be very wary of an over-dependence on rote learning.

'Learning number facts and procedures' could suggest that a key approach to maths involves memorising facts and procedures. There is evidence to support this interpretation (for example, Ofsted 2008). Again, an over-reliance on memory, 'learning by heart', is ineffective for any learner, but is very detrimental for many more than officialdom might acknowledge, particularly those with learning difficulties. There is further evidence that maths education in the UK is seriously ineffective for around 25 per cent of learners (Rashid and Brookes 2010; Chinn 2013). This leads into the part about performing maths tasks mechanically and without confidence and probably infers that the learner lacks an ability to appraise answers for validity and correctness. The skill of estimation (Chapter 22) is not a natural one for many learners. This vital life-skill area of maths has, therefore to be taught, and in an empathetic way that matches the learner's cognitive (thinking) style.

Chapter summary

Some of the factors that can create barriers to learning mathematics

an ability to work with symbols   maths vocabulary

working memory

short-term memory   speed of processing

long-term memory   sequencing   reversing

cognitive style   anxiety

generalising/patterns

BUT they interlink (for example, anxiety depresses working memory)

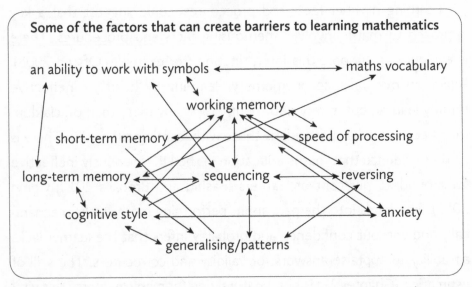

Figure 1.1 Some of the factors that can create barriers to learning mathematics

It's complicated!

Chapter 2

Why Children May Not Learn Maths

When I am lecturing to teachers from across the UK and abroad, the answer to my question, 'At what age are enough children giving up on maths in class for it to be noticeable?' varies, of course, but the most frequent answer I get is 'seven years old'. Then I meet 18-year-old students who know less maths than we expect a 10-year-old to know... despite having endured some 13 years of maths lessons. Amazingly, impressively, many still try, often spurred on by the reality that to enter the higher or further education course of their choice, someone has decided, often quite arbitrarily, that it is 'important' to pass a specified exam at a specified level/grade. For example, without maths there can be no training as a designer or artist.

The percentage for whom this is a problem is probably around 20 to 25 per cent; of these some will be dyscalculic, some dyslexic, some dyspraxic, some all three. It seems obvious to conclude that the way they are being taught is not working for them.

So what factors are blocking learning? If it starts at seven years old, we can't blame algebra, or fractions, or even division, though these topics probably finish off a lot of children later when they appear in the curriculum. It could be anxiety. That would be very bad, to have children as young as seven being anxious about maths to a level where they want to give up. Sadly, it happens.

Basically, I don't know a definitive answer to this question and I feel that I should. However, my preliminary research suggests that there are a number of factors, including the following:

- Having to do maths calculations quickly.

- (Rote) learning facts and procedures (without understanding them).

- The extremely judgemental nature of maths. An answer is right, or it is wrong. The issue here is that failure rarely motivates, especially over-exposure to overt failure.

- The inconsistencies in early arithmetic confuse children, making bigger challenges on memory and blurring concepts.

- Being asked to do tasks that are beyond the capacity of the child's working and short-term memories.

- The vocabulary and language of early maths is often everyday vocabulary and language, but then it is used in a maths setting (for example, 'take away' means 'subtraction'). This is confusing, bad for communication and is an example of inconsistencies. This situation is exacerbated by the extensive use of symbols in maths.

(For a longer discussion on these factors see Chinn 2017a or Chinn and Ashcroft 2017.)

The interactions and combinations of these factors and their relative impact on the individual will differ from child to child.

As ever in teaching and learning, communication is critical. In maths, teachers are not merely communicating facts and information, they are communicating concepts. There are a number of essential elements for communication, including the following:

- Short-term memory. If instructions or information are given out at a level or quantity that exceeds the short-term memory capacity of the child, the information will not be remembered by the child. When short-term memory forgets an item or items, it forgets completely. Thus, the communication has failed at the first hurdle.

- Working memory. This is the memory that is particularly important for mental arithmetic. Assuming the pupil has enough short-term memory capacity to remember the question, they then need to use working memory to perform the calculation. If the number of steps they use or plan to use exceed their working memory capacity, then they will fail at the task. If that makes them anxious then the problem gets worse, because anxiety can depress the capacity of working memory even further.

- Consistency is reassuring. It makes the general background of life secure, so that a few new experiences can be dealt with. Without that consistency, and the security it brings, learning will be less effective. For example, fractions give the impression of inconsistency if they are not explained carefully, in the vocabulary used, the hidden symbols (especially ÷), in procedures and in number sense.

- Having to do maths calculations quickly can challenge children with special needs, who often are slower at processing information. This creates more anxiety, which results in less working memory capacity, more failure, more anxiety, less motivation and the cycle spirals.

- Committing basic facts and procedures to long-term memory. This seems to be a particular problem with the times tables facts. I hear too many people use the very illogical statement, to the effect that, 'If I learned them and all my friends learned them, why can't you?' Again, I do not know exactly why this task is so very difficult for some children (and adults), though I have some ideas, but I do know that it *is* difficult to the level of being impossible for some, or certainly unproductive in the time spent on the task compared to the gains made. Learning times tables is a part of maths that parents feel confident to do with their child. This task, unlike many topics in maths, has not been changed by curriculum 'innovations'. It is consistent in its content! There is a way to deal with the problem with a mathematically and conceptually productive approach (see Chapter 11). Another of my surveys of the teachers who attend my training sessions and lectures is about the percentage of pupils who know these facts at age 10 or 11 years. The responses are rarely lower than 50 per cent and can reach as high as 70 per cent. Once more, if the pupil does not know the answers, that is more experience of failure, more demotivation.

- The vocabulary of early maths is discussed in Chapter 9, but the problem continues as the maths progresses, for example, 1/2, 1/3 and 1/4, which are the first fractions that children will meet and meet most frequently. They have names that are exceptions to the later pattern of 'fourth, fifth, sixth, seventh, etc.'. They are not, 'twoth and threeth' and they can be confused with ordinal numbers, as in, 'coming fifth in the race'.

It may be that teachers and parents have not recognised and acknowledged these factors with the consequence that the learning environment for children is not efficacious. It is a not uncommon occurrence in life that, just because something makes sense to one person (themselves), it automatically makes sense to everyone else. They may think, 'If I can learn these facts, as everyone did in my school days, then why can't you?'

Chapter 3

Maths Anxiety

Beyond any other school subject, maths anxiety is a big problem. You can buy books on maths anxiety, but not on history anxiety or art anxiety. Maths is a subject that creates anxiety in too many children and adults. Closely linked to this anxiety is a fear of negative evaluation: being told that you are wrong. Few people find that encouraging. So, it is not surprising that one of the main consequences of anxiety is that people give up on maths.

Our, Western, society colludes with this situation, people say to children, 'Don't worry, I could never do maths' or 'Why do we need maths anyway?' Added to this is the situation that too many parents find themselves unable to help their children with any maths beyond the times table facts (and many adults are unable to remember all of those). We need to remember that apart from parents' own insecurities about maths, many of the methods that are now taught in schools were not the methods taught when they went to school. Children do not respond well to, 'I wasn't taught that method, this is the way I was taught.' They are then confused by a different method and don't ask for help again.

It's not just when doing maths, it's often the anticipation of doing maths. Recent neurological research has shown that the area of the brain that is activated when maths anxious children are anticipating doing maths is the same bit that is activated when anticipating physical harm. The anxiety is a neurological reality.

I did a large survey into maths anxiety in 2084 secondary students (Chinn 2009) selecting 20 situations/demands that I thought would create anxiety. The highest anxiety scores were for:

- taking an end-of-term maths examination (top item for all ages, male and female and dyslexic students)

- waiting to hear your score on a maths test

- answering long division questions without a calculator

- having to work out answers to maths questions quickly.

The pressure of doing maths quickly discriminates against people who are slow processors.

Some other factors contributing to maths anxiety are:

- a poor understanding of maths, often resulting in helplessness (and often at the very basic level)

- a poor long-term memory for maths facts and procedures (and no effective way to compensate)

- inappropriate instruction (for example, instruction that does not acknowledge memory issues, long-term, short-term and working and lack of support from visual images)

- badly designed work tasks, for example, with content beyond the learner's capabilities or over-designed, overcrowded worksheets (and over-facing the student with too many questions)

- the pace of the curriculum, moving on before the pupil has grasped the topic. (There is a need for built-in frequent revisits and refreshers.)

- constant experience of underachievement or failure (the student becomes 'helpless', thinking, 'I'm no good at this, never will be and you can't help me')

- teachers' attitudes, parents' attitudes, society's attitudes, none of which acknowledge the learning needs of the child ('this worked for me, so it should work for you')

- the pressure of having to do maths quickly. We should ask ourselves, 'What is the rush?' 'Where did this culture come from?'

- the extremely judgemental nature of maths, that is, answers are almost always judged as 'right' or 'wrong' thus generating a fear of negative evaluation (instead of, for example, 'That was pretty close, you just made a place value error here.' In fact, error analysis can tell you why a child is failing, going beyond just telling them they are 'WRONG').

If teachers and parents address these problems, then anxiety is going to be reduced and, maybe, even pre-empted.

Chapter 4

Cognition and Meta-Cognition in Maths

Maths curricula across the world seem to be moving to some similarities in pedagogy. One of these is that the curriculum must encourage flexible thinking and meta-cognition (or 'thinking about how and what you are thinking'). There seems to be some consensus, even if only in principle, that there should be less emphasis on the use of formulas/algorithms.

Usiskin (1998, p.36) listed the benefits and attractions of algorithms (formulas):

- *Power:* An algorithm applies to a class of problems.

- *Reliability and accuracy:* Done correctly, an algorithm always provides the correct answer.

- *Speed:* An algorithm proceeds directly to the answer.

- *A record:* A paper and pencil algorithm provides a record of how the answer was determined.

The seductive power of algorithms is enhanced by the many students who collude with teachers in accepting an over-emphasis on the use of algorithms. For example, the mantra for dividing by a fraction, 'Turn upside down and multiply', is accepted as saving a lot of agony and effort in trying to understand the logic behind the procedure.

There is a problem here for students who do not have reliable long-term mathematical memories. Formulas, procedures and accurate and swift recall of facts will lead to a version of success in number work for those children with strong mathematical memories, but even in this case, society needs problem solvers as well as computationally adept pupils (particularly when calculators and computers are readily available). And brains are designed to forget, particularly when the topic is not 'topped up' in memory. I firmly believe that understanding maths enhances the memory for maths. Singapore, a country with a strong reputation for success in maths, overtly encourages meta-cognition.

I was involved in research into thinking (cognitive) style in maths with two colleagues in the USA in the mid-1980s (Bath, Chinn and Knox 1986). Our literature search showed that two styles of thinking seemed to be recognised and *that good problem solvers needed to use the appropriate thinking style at different stages in problem solving*. We labelled our version of the two styles as 'Inchworm' and 'Grasshopper' and researched the practical implications for teaching maths.

Grasshoppers are holistic, flexible and intuitive. They have very good number and operation senses. They resist documenting their methods. Grasshoppers are answer-oriented. Inchworms are formulaic, procedural, sequential and literal in their interpretation of numbers. They need to document and want only one way to solve problems. Inchworms are procedure-oriented (see Table 4.1).

It is possible that some educators underestimate the impact of this concept. It seems obvious that the way that learners think will be a very critical factor in the way they learn and the way they are taught. The concept of meta-cognition has been recognised as a major contributor to success in teaching and learning. The National Research Council of the USA published their findings and research in *How People Learn* (Bransford, Brown and Cocking 2000). They summarised their research in just three key findings, the third of which is: 'The teaching of metacognitive skills should be integrated into the curriculum in a variety of subject areas' (p.21).

Table 4.1 Cognitive styles of the inchworm and grasshopper

	Inchworm	Grasshopper
I Analysing and identifying the problem	1. Focuses on the parts and details; separates.	1. Tends to overview; holistic; puts together.
	2. Looks at the numbers and facts to select a relevant formula or procedure.	2. Looks at the numbers and facts to estimate an answer or restrict the range of the answer; controlled exploration.
II Solving the problem	3. Formula, procedure orientated.	3. Answer orientated.
	4. Constrained focus; uses a single method.	4. Flexible focusing; methods change.
	5. Works in serially ordered steps, usually forward (rifle).	5. Often works back from a trial answer; multi-method (shot gun).
	6. Uses numbers exactly as given.	6. Adjusts, breaks down/ builds up numbers to make an easier calculation.
	7. More comfortable with paper and pen; documents the method.	7. Rarely documents the method; performs calculation mentally.
III Checking and evaluating	8. Unlikely to check or evaluate the answer; if check is done, uses the same procedure or method.	8. Likely to appraise and evaluate answer against original estimate; checks by an alternate method.
	9. Often does not understand procedures or values of numbers; works mechanically.	9. Has good understanding of the numbers, methods and relationships.

Source: Chinn and Ashcroft (2017). Reproduced with kind permission from Wiley.

Hattie's (2009) highly regarded study of the research into what is effective in education found that meta-cognitive strategies were very effective in improving learning. He also mentions within this context the use of self-questioning and states that 'the more varied the instructional strategies throughout a lesson, the more students are influenced' (p.218). I am often asked if too many strategies are explained, will they cause confusion. My answer is a succinct 'No', but the way that variety is presented is very critical as to whether, or not, it is beneficial (see also later).

Uncertain learners like the security of the familiar, even if the familiar is not all that successful. Consistency is a key factor in motivation. Teachers may have to do the hard sell on that alternative method.

There are some potential consequences, in terms of being successful at maths, that are linked to the two thinking styles. If the learner is at either extreme of the cognitive style spectrum then they will be at risk. It is possible to survive maths as an 'extreme' inchworm, but there are some essential prerequisite skills that are needed to make this an effective style, for example a good long-term memory for sequential information and a good working memory. It is less likely that a grasshopper will survive secondary school maths, particularly when documentation is essential. A grasshopper mathematician is likely to be successful at 'life maths', but probably not as an accounts clerk.

Some maths curricula encourage pupils to share their different methods and encourage teachers to present different methods for solving problems. Again, this will require good sales techniques from teachers, because some pupils will just not want to buy into different methods because they think one method is enough and two or more will be confusing (and, in their opinion, unnecessary!) However, each method should illustrate another facet of the problem and, even if the pupil doesn't adopt the new method, an exposure to a different way of perceiving a problem should be beneficial in developing understanding of a concept. Plus, there will be a range of needs in that group of pupils.

However, there are persuasive reasons why it is beneficial for learners to be able to draw on *both* thinking styles, maybe even during the solving of a single question. A problem-solving sequence might be: start with the overviewing skills of the grasshopper, move onto the documenting and procedural skills of the inchworm and finally check the answer using the appraising skills of the grasshopper. Then there is the situation that some questions and topics lend themselves more to one thinking style than the other, for example, mental arithmetic tends to be a better experience for grasshoppers, whilst algebra is more inchworm friendly, primarily in the way it is taught.

The ethos of the classroom is another key factor in encouraging or discouraging flexible thinking styles. If learners are encouraged to explore different methods and their efforts are praised and appreciated (children are adept at spotting false praise) then they will generate a learning culture of flexible thinking. This goal also requires a risk-taking ethos in the classroom where pupils can be wrong without losing motivation.

Pupils can be encouraged to share and discuss different methods, but, again, teachers must be aware that there is a need to manage those extreme inchworms who may be confused by too much choice. Valuing different approaches will encourage flexibility. The maths culture of answering quickly will be counter-productive for these goals. If we are encouraging pupils to read, overview, digest, analyse and comprehend questions, to use meta-cognition, then the culture of speedy answers may discourage them from doing that.

There is almost always more than one way to solve a maths problem, however simple the problem seems to be. Children will become better problem solvers if they can think of 'another way' to solve a problem. This will also help them check their answers and become more confident with those answers. Adults can still learn this skill. Learning to leave the old skill behind for a time while you learn another, almost contradictory, skill is hard for any sports player. It's hard to do in academic activities, too. The old, safe and secure methods are just that, safe and secure. In the early stages of learning, a new skill may appear unappealingly inefficient. Hopefully that changes and the new skill can take its place alongside the old skill.

Finally, it should be noted that there may be some inchworms and some grasshoppers whose thinking style is terminal and totally impervious to change, however skilled the teacher. Then the teacher needs to remember the adage, 'Teach the subject as it is to the child as she is.'

Maths skills and cognitive style

Three key grasshopper skills an inchworm should adopt:

1. Inter-relating numbers and the operations, for example, seeing 9 as 1 less than 10, seeing 5 as half of 10.

2. Overviewing any problem, for example, reading to the end before starting or getting a feel of what the answer might be.

3. Appraising their answer.

Three key inchworm skills a grasshopper should adopt:

1. Explaining their methods.

2. Documenting their methods.

3. Accepting algebra! (It can confirm their reasoning.)

Chapter 5

Key Numbers

This could be a variation on the infamous philosophy of the pigs in George Orwell's *Animal Farm*, 'All numbers are equal, but some are more equal than others.' (It could also be about 'equal' meaning different things to different people.)

The overwhelmingly most frequently occurring numbers that are used for coinage and money systems, internationally, are 1, 2, 5, 10, 20, 50, 100 and so on. The multiplication facts that are most frequently and reliably remembered by children and adults are 1x, 2x, 5x, and 10x.

The base 10 system that we use is based on counting fingers. Again, the key numbers are 1 finger, 2 hands, 5 fingers per hand and 10 fingers altogether.

Professor Brian Butterworth's theory for dyscalculia has two pre-requisite skills that distinguish a dyscalculic. One of these is subitising, the ability to look at a quantity of randomly arranged dots (1 to 5 dots) and know how many are there. This is about a sense of quantity and the numbers associated with a quantity.

Look at the two clusters of dots below and say how many are there. Do not count, use your judgement.

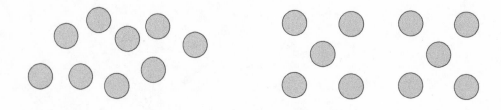

The first cluster is 9, the second is 10. The pattern for the second cluster makes the appraisal more accurate, and that appraisal will be more consistent.

These, inter-relating, patterns will be used throughout this book to provide a consistent visual image for quantity, based on 1, 2, 5 and 10.

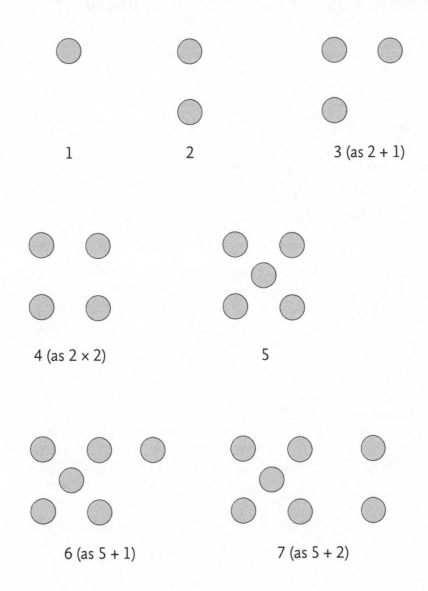

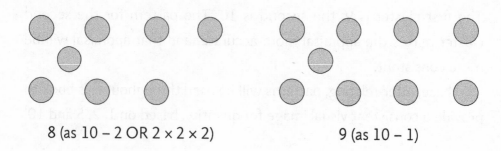

8 (as 10 – 2 OR 2 × 2 × 2)   9 (as 10 – 1)

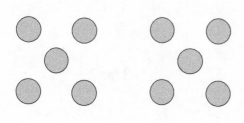

10 (as 2 × 5)

Chapter 6

Early Number Experiences

Number (and operation) concepts are unequivocally fundamental to progress. Get the foundations secure, not just in long-term memory as facts, but as interlinking concepts.

I sometimes visit bookshops to browse the books about numbers that are targeted at young children. Often, in fact, usually, they are more about design than content. Sadly, this observation applies to some books that target older learners, too, where the inclusion of drawings of cute animals in clustered groups blur the concept of number that they are supposed to illustrate. I realise that meerkats may not naturally cluster themselves in manageable and identifiable patterns in real life, but then the illustrations in maths books are rarely drawn to look like real life anyway.

I believe that two factors are influential here. One is the dominant power of the first learning experience (Buswell and Judd 1925) and the other is the negative influence of apparent inconsistencies in many of the aspects of learning. However, we must remember that consistency may take different manifestations for different children. For example, two ways could be used to represent numbers visually:

A linear arrangement:

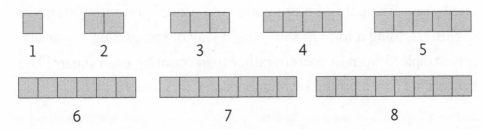

Which could include a differentiation to show the contribution of 5:

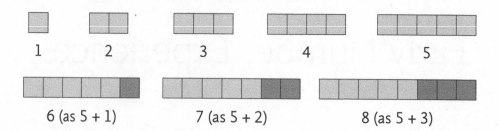

1   2   3   4   5

6 (as 5 + 1)   7 (as 5 + 2)   8 (as 5 + 3)

The second representation is as a pattern (see also Chapter 4):

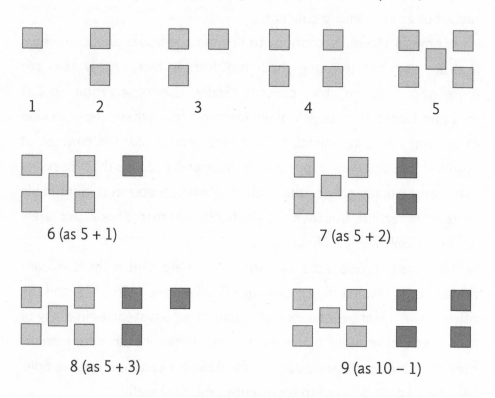

1   2   3   4   5

6 (as 5 + 1)   7 (as 5 + 2)

8 (as 5 + 3)   9 (as 10 − 1)

The linear presentation may suit the children who like to count, often one by one. The pattern presentation is a way of presenting numbers in clusters, using a form of subitising, a way of recognising a quantity, for example, 5 from its pattern rather than counting each square. The clusters are based on the key numbers of 1, 2, 5 and 10.

The squares may not be as attractive as the cartoons of worms or meerkats or ladybirds, but they can be used to show, in an uncluttered way, the relationships between numbers. For example, the patterns

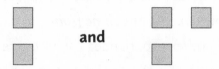

can be used to show that 3 is more than 2, that 3 is bigger than 2, that 3 is one more than 2, that 3 is 2 + 1, that 2 is one less than 3, that 2 is 3 take away 1 (and the 'take away' is a literal interpretation if the square is actually taken away). Even for such basic relationships the vocabulary can be confusingly varied. I could have said, '1 is subtracted from 3' or '3 subtract 1' (thereby changing the order for the digits).

The two patterns

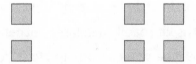

can be used to show that 4 is 'double 2', 'two times two', 'two plus two' (which is repeated addition and thus linked to multiplication, 2 × 2) or that 2 is half of 4 (showing division as the inverse of multiplication).

There are learning/teaching implications for this approach. The patterns, both the visual patterns and the symbol patterns, can be used at a range of levels. They are developmental. They take a basic concept and can be used to develop that into other concepts. This could be seen as sowing the seeds of maths development, setting down the roots for future growth, there to be referred back to time and again as the maths develops. For example, the question, 'Is it bigger or smaller?' encourages children to appraise their answers in a reasonably low-stress way, using an aspect of estimation. The relationships between 2 and 4 can set the foundations for repeated multiplication (×4 as ×2×2 and ×8 as ×2×2×2 or ×2³), for division and for the doubles facts.

For early maths it helps to know where the maths is going; for later maths it helps to know where it has come from.

For these early number experiences the visual representations are used to develop a sense of number and how numbers and operations inter-relate. This is using single-digit numbers, but that will progress to become two-digit numbers (and beyond).

Materials and manipulatives

As a teacher of physics, in the early days of my teaching career, it would have been bizarre not to use apparatus to set up experiments to demonstrate concepts, even at Advanced level. So, I find the use of materials to illustrate maths concepts quite a natural thing to do. I believe that every maths classroom should have a maths kit readily available, either in a cupboard or in a toolbox of the type you can buy in Do It Yourself stores, so that the contents are ready to use when explaining some maths process or concept that a pupil or pupils find confusing. Match the material to the concept and the vocabulary and, when possible, to the learner(s), using the materials and language alongside the maths symbols, so that the link is made between the 'bricks' and the 'numbers'.

There are many examples of materials being used throughout this book.

Before we move to the next development, two-digit numbers, I want to introduce a structure that will be used with each topic in the following chapters. The key learning factors will be considered for each topic. These are:

- vocabulary and language

- images, symbols and concepts

- the relevance of the topic/concept to developing maths skills

- meta-cognition (thinking about how and what you are thinking)

- things to do and practise.

Chapter 7

Two-Digit Numbers

Two-digit numbers start at 10 and end at 99.

Vocabulary and language

The English language does not offer consistency for the two-digit numbers, particularly from 10 to 19. This must be very confusing for young children when they meet them for the first time. The vocabulary does not support the pattern of the symbols.

The words for the first two-digit numbers after 10 are exceptions: eleven and twelve. The numbers that then take us towards 20, the teen numbers, suggest an order that is the reverse to what we write with digits, for example, we say 'fourteen' which hints at 4 and 10, but we write 14: 10 and 4. As well as the vocabulary, there is a very sophisticated concept here, the concept of place value.

Images, symbols and concepts

The symbols for fourteen are 14, a 1 and a 4 in a specific order. Change the order and 14 becomes 41, forty-one. There are two places where we could place the digits:

_____ _____ which can be 1 4 or 4 1

If we write 1 in the first place and 4 in the second place then that 14 is fourteen, 1 ten and 4 ones.

If we write 4 in the first place and 1 in the second place then that 41 is forty-one, 4 tens and 1 one.

If we use coins as our kinaesthetic/visual images, then fourteen, 14, is one 10p coin and four 1p coins and forty-one, 41, is four 10p coins and one 1p coin:

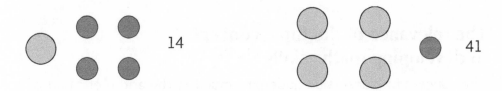

14

41

So, the *place* where we write the digits (relative to each other) in the number determines the *value* they represent. In this example, 1 can represent 1 ten or it can represent 1 one. 4 can represent 4 ones or 4 tens. This is the logic of *place value.*

One key reason for this being a big problem is that this first experience that children have of place value as a concept, a very vital and pervasive concept, is not supported by the vocabulary.

Things improve in the twenties, thirties, forties and on. For example, we say forty-five and write 45. Sadly, we don't say 4 tens and 5. We learn to understand that the '-ty' is a distortion of 'ten'.

Another problem for some children is discriminating (aurally) the sounds of 'thirteen' and 'thirty', 'fourteen' and 'forty', and even 'twenty' and 'twelve', but if teachers and parents are aware of the potential for confusion then they can guard against it, possibly by using visuals or materials (such as coins or base 10 materials/Dienes blocks).

Bead strings and coins are good materials for supporting the concept of place value as are base 10 blocks. The effective strategy is to show the materials alongside the numbers and to connect these and to talk the learner through the relevance of the illustration.

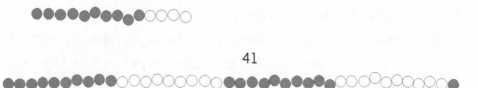

14

41

The relevance of the topic/concept to developing maths skills

The concept of place value underpins much of the arithmetic part of mathematics. For example, addition and subtraction, multiplying and dividing by tens, hundreds, thousands and so on, and decimals. As well as developing a flexible understanding of numbers, for example 'seeing' that 46 is 30 + 16 and that 9 is one less than 10, learners need to understand the role of zero in place value. Roman numerals do not include a zero. Zero was introduced when the Hindu-Arabic system of number entered the UK some seven hundred years ago.

Two of the major goals for teachers are to develop a clear understanding of place value in their pupils and to wean them off counting in ones.

Chapter 8

Moving from One-Digit to Two-Digit Numbers, from Two-Digit to Three-Digit Numbers…and Back

The process of 'crossing' the tens, for example, from 9 to 10 (and the hundreds, for example, from 99 to 100, and so on for the thousands, etc.), is one of the fundamental concepts of maths. It is a very important part of place value.

Vocabulary and language

'Crossing' the tens means crossing from 10 ones to 1 ten. This is sometimes known as 'trading' or as 'carrying' or as 're-naming' when doing addition problems.

When the 'crossing' is going back, it is crossing from 1 ten to 10 ones. This can be called 're-grouping' or 'decomposing' or 'borrowing' or 'trading'. (My preferred word for both crossings is 'trading'.) This is used in some subtraction problems.

Images, symbols and concepts

The images used below are coins. Note that the symbols, the digits, are written next to the images. You must link the visual to the symbol.

Remember coins are not proportional in size to the values they represent.

THE TASK

When we count up to, and then past 10, we move from a one-digit number to a two-digit number where one digit represents tens and the other represents ones according to the place they hold in the number.

Let's start at 8 and count up to 12 and let's look at how it works by using 1p and 10p coins:

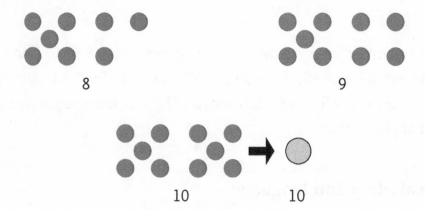

When we reach ten, we can exchange to ten 1p coins for one 10p coin. So, as we cross the tens there is an exchange (or trade). Sometimes in maths this is called re-naming or re-grouping.

Now as we count onwards, 11, 12, 13, the 10p coin represents, of course, the ten, and the 1p coins represent the ones.

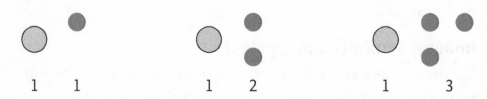

Another exchange happens as we cross the tens and count from 19 to 20:

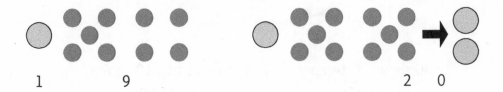

1   9   2   0

The zero, 0, in 20 tells us that there are zero ones. It also keeps the tens-digit in the correct place, where the tens-digits should be. If the zero, 0, was not there then we would have just 2.

The next exchange, the next time we cross the tens, is from 29 to 30:

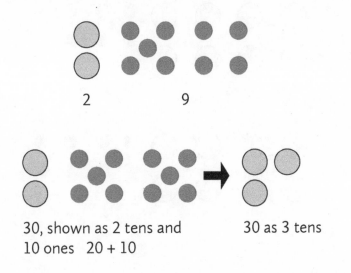

2   9

30, shown as 2 tens and   30 as 3 tens
10 ones 20 + 10

When we count backwards the exchange is reversed; it is the opposite procedure. We change one 10p coin for ten 1p coins. For example, it helps to 'see' or visualise 30 as three 10p coins and then as two 10p coins plus ten 1p coins, that is as 20 + 10:

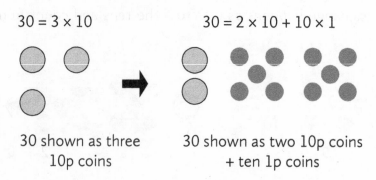

$$30 = 3 \times 10$$

$$30 = 2 \times 10 + 10 \times 1$$

30 shown as three
10p coins

30 shown as two 10p coins
+ ten 1p coins

Then we can count back in ones and take away one 1p coin each time.

The same concept applies when we move from two-digit to three-digit numbers. So, for the sequence, 98, 99, 100, 101 we have:

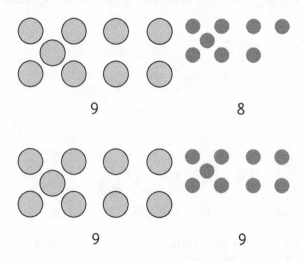

Now we get a double cross (!). The next one we add takes the 9 ones to 10 ones, which crosses the tens and we trade the 10 ones (1p coins) for 1 ten (a 10p coin). That makes ten 10p coins so we trade again, but this time we trade ten 10p coins for one £1 coin (100p).

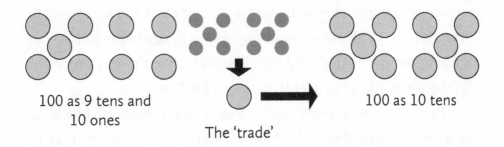

100 as 9 tens and   The 'trade'   100 as 10 tens
      10 ones

These visual images should be demonstrated first with the coins and backed up with discussion and diagnostic questioning to ensure that the concept is understood.

The relevance of the topic/concept to developing maths skills

Counting on builds the foundation for addition and counting back builds the foundation for subtraction.

The concepts here are place value and 'trading'. Place value underpins our number system. Trading will be a key concept when we move onto addition and subtraction. It will be used again in other topics.

All the demonstrations above can and should be demonstrated with base 10 blocks (which can be bought online from a range of suppliers).

Meta-cognition (thinking about how and what you are thinking)

The learner should be encouraged to articulate their perceptions of these demonstrations. Diagnostic questioning may well help this, for example, 'Can you explain what is happening with the coins when you show me the sequence 38, 39, 40, 41?'

Can they now demonstrate 998, 999, 1000 (a £10 note)?

This is also reinforcing an understanding of coins and notes, which, unlike the base 10 blocks are not proportional in size to the values they represent. (In Australia, the $2 coin is smaller than the 1$ coin! In the USA the dime, 10c, is smaller than the nickel, 5c!)

If these concepts were demonstrated with base 10 blocks as well as with coins, then that 'base 10' part of the concept may be demonstrated more directly since the sizes of these materials are in proportion to the values they represent.

Things to do and practise

Practise crossing the tens, both ways, for a range of examples, such as 49 to 50 and 50 to 49, and 79 to 80 and 80 to 79. Do this with coins and symbols, base 10 blocks and symbols and then only symbols.

Practise counting on in tens, starting from numbers such as 17 (27, 37, 47...), 14 (24, 34, 44, 54...), 35 (45, 55, 65, 75...), or 48 (58, 68, 78...). Do a similar practice exercise counting backwards.

Do similar exercises for 197 to 202, 499 to 503 and 789 to 801.

Can the learner extend the concept to 999 to 1001?

Ask the learner to point to the tens-digit in numbers such as 2961, 641 and 1007 and then do similar exercises to point out hundreds and thousands digits.

Encourage the learner to articulate their thinking as they carry out the tasks (meta-cognition again).

Chapter 9

Basic Facts for Addition and Subtraction

These are the 'facts' for the addition of any one-digit number or 10 to another one-digit number or 10. That is, from 0 + 0 to 10 + 10. They are probably known as 'basic' facts because, if students know them, they can work out all other whole number additions.

There is an equivalent collection of basic facts for subtraction, from 20 – 10 to 0 – 0.

One of the most useful things about these basic facts is that they can be used to work out a fact that may have been forgotten, or to check it, if the learner is not 100 per cent sure of the answer (and preferable to using finger counting). These basic facts interlink. For example, if you know that 10 + 7 is 17, and you understand that 9 + 7 will give you an answer that is smaller and smaller by 1, so then, from 10 + 7 = 17 you can get 9 + 7 = 16, without counting 7 onto 9, or indeed retrieving the fact from long-term memory. From 10 + 7 you can extrapolate to 100 + 70, 1000 + 700 and so on (and thus re-visit place value).

So, if pupils can use number skills to work out more facts and answers from the ones that they do remember, then it is worth considering which facts are the most useful to memorise.

Vocabulary and language

There are several words that are used for the addition symbol + and the subtraction symbol –. Learners need to be familiar with the words used for these symbols.

So, for example, 7 + 6 can be said as:

7 plus 6

7 add 6

7 and 6

7 and 6 more

7 more than 6

the total for 6 and 7 is

and 13 – 6 can be said as:

13 minus 6

13 take away 6

What is the difference between 13 and 6?

13 subtract 6

What is 6 less than 13?

Images, symbols and concepts

The images and/or materials that could be used to illustrate these facts include counters, coins, Cuisenaire rods, base 10 blocks and number lines. Creative minds could find many other resources, such as sweets or rulers.

The concepts here are that:

addition and subtraction are reverse 'operations' so,

the two operations are linked and thus,

the number facts involved interlink, e.g. 7 + 6 = 13

13 – 7 = 6.

There can be an interaction between the vocabulary used and the manipulatives that are used. For example, subtraction can be implied with the words:

'What is the difference between 7 and 4?' or 'From 7 take away 4'.

The first can be modelled with Stern blocks, which can be compared to show the 'difference'.

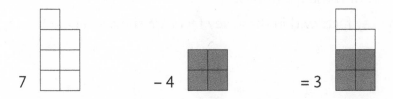

The second can be modelled with counters.

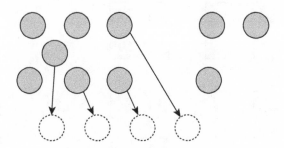

THE TASK

So, which are the most useful facts to learn? Part of the way we find the answer to that question is by asking a second question, 'Which facts are most useful for working out other facts and doing other maths?'

Three of the most useful sets of facts are:

the doubles, e.g. 7 + 7

the number bonds for 10, e.g. 6 + 4   2 + 8

and the 10 plus a single digit, e.g.   10 + 3

Effort should be focused on memorising these facts. Images (and materials) should help in memorising them.

Doubles

The answers to the 'doubles' are always even numbers, 2, 4, 6, 8, 10, 12, 14, 16, 18 and 20. The patterns used in Chapters 5 and 6 may help. They are used again here to maintain consistency in the patterns used to represent these quantities.

The key facts within these key facts are shown in bold here:

$1 + 1 = 2$

$2 + 2 = 4$

$3 + 3 = 6$

$4 + 4 = 8$

$5 + 5 = 10$

5 + 5 = 10 is a truly key pattern and fact (see following page).

6 + 6 = 12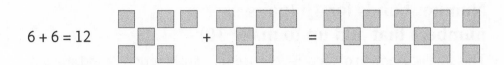

Note that 6 is shown as 5 + 1. The pattern then shows 6 + 6 as 5 + 5 + 1 + 1. A similar pattern works for 7 + 7, 8 + 8 and 9 + 9. (It compares to 2 + 2, 3 + 3 and 4 + 4.)

7 + 7 = 14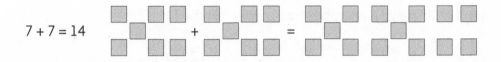

Set up the patterns with the materials of choice for the remaining 'doubles'.

It is useful to learn the doubles as subtraction facts, too.

$$18 - 9 = 9$$
$$16 - 8 = 8$$
$$14 - 7 = 7$$
$$12 - 6 = 6$$
$$10 - 5 = 5$$
$$8 - 4 = 4$$
$$6 - 3 = 3$$
$$4 - 2 = 2$$
$$2 - 1 = 1$$

Doubles can be extended to develop 'doubles +/- 1' and 'shared doubles', for example:

5 + 5 leads to   5 + 6 and 6 + 5   and   4 + 5 and 5 + 4   and (shared) 4 + 6 and 6 + 4

Number bonds for 10 (pairs of numbers that add up to make 10)

This small collection of facts is very useful in arithmetic. A good starting point is our hands. We have 2 hands with 5 fingers on each hand, a total of 10 fingers (thumbs are included as fingers in maths).

A bead string could be a suitable manipulative to use here. It emphasises that there are always ten beads, none fall off, none jump on. This conservation of number is another example of breaking down (and building up) a number from other numbers.

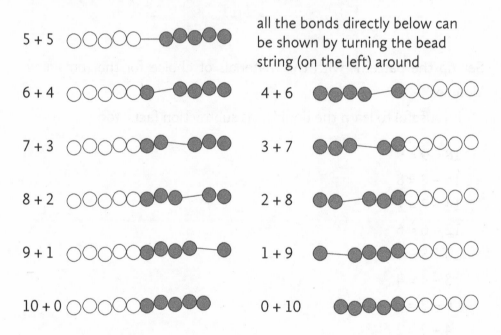

all the bonds directly below can be shown by turning the bead string (on the left) around

It is useful to learn the number bonds for 10 as subtraction facts, too:

$10 - 0 = 10$
$10 - 1 = 9$
$10 - 2 = 8$
$10 - 3 = 7$
$10 - 4 = 6$

$10 - 5 = 5$

$10 - 6 = 4$

$10 - 7 = 3$

$10 - 8 = 2$

$10 - 9 = 1$

$10 - 10 = 0$

Adding a single-digit number to 10

This could be demonstrated with coins. The constant presence of the 10p coins emphasises that the tens digit does not change. The pattern for the ones digits is the same as used for counting from 1 to 9. Only the first four examples are illustrated with coins. Remember that the vocabulary (for example, thirteen) for these numbers does not support a pattern that matches the digits and their order in the number.

$10 + 1 = 11$

$10 + 2 = 12$

$10 + 3 = 13$

$10 + 4 = 14$

It may be worth showing the sequence for 20 to 29 to illustrate how the vocabulary matches the concept in a more helpful way.

These facts can be extended by considering and comparing the outcomes of adding 10 and adding 9. Adding 9 instead of 10 will result in an answer that is 1 less in comparison, for example:

$10 + 4 = 14$ $9 + 4 = 13$

$10 + 6 = 16$ $9 + 6 = 15$

$10 + 8 = 18$ $9 + 8 = 17$

This can be used as an exercise in estimation and in the use of the question, 'Is it bigger or smaller?'

Motivation may be enhanced when the number square is filled in with the families of facts from above as well as adding 0, adding 1 or adding 2 (these are quick to count on if necessary). Very few facts remain. Try it.

+	0	1	2	3	4	5	6	7	8	9	10
0											
1											
2											
3											
4											
5											
6											
7											
8											
9											
10											

The relevance of the topic/concept to developing maths skills

From the doubles, the fact 5 + 5 = 10 is a truly key fact in that pattern/ collection. It is the foundation of our number system. We have 2 hands, there are 5 fingers on each hand and 2 × 5 is 10. Each finger is *one* and together we have *ten* fingers. We then extend this idea to ten lots of ten... a *hundred*, 100, ten lots of a hundred are a *thousand*, 1000. The number of digits in each of these numbers is increasing.

For ones: 1 digit

For tens: 2 digits

For hundreds: 3 digits

For thousands: 4 digits

For millions: 7 digits

The value a digit represents depends on the place it takes in the number. So, in 412, the 2 is '2 ones'. In 8627, the 2 is '2 tens'. In 3251, the 2 is '2 hundreds'. In 2095, the 2 is '2 thousands'. In this collection of examples, the 2 becomes a number that is ten times (10×) bigger with each place it moves to the left in the number. This concept will be referred to many times as the maths progresses.

This using the same digit to represent different values, depending on its place in a number, is not true for Roman numerals, where 1 is I, 10 is X, 100 is C and 1000 is M.

For the number bonds for 10:

These can be extended, by using place value, to the number bonds for 100.

0 + 100	10 + 90	20 + 80	30 + 70	40 + 60	50 + 50
100 + 0	90 + 10	80 + 20	70 + 30	60 + 40	

Again, using place value, the pattern extends to the decimal number bonds for 1.

$$0 + 1 \quad 0.1 + 0.9 \quad 0.2 + 0.8 \quad 0.3 + 0.7 \quad 0.4 + 0.6 \quad 0.5 + 0.5$$

$$1 + 0 \quad 0.9 + 0.1 \quad 0.8 + 0.2 \quad 0.7 + 0.3 \quad 0.6 + 0.4$$

And this applies for 0.1 and 1000 and, as a good generalisation should do, to any power of 10.

Number bonds for 10 are also very useful when adding columns of numbers, using them to 'cast out tens', a procedure that will be described in the next chapter.

Presenting the bonds as

$$6 + 4 = \boxed{} \quad \text{and} \quad 6 + \boxed{} = 10$$

and $6 + 4 = y$ and $6 + q = 10$

introduces algebra.

These key number bonds and the others derived from them are used in addition, subtraction multiplication and division problems.

Meta-cognition (thinking about how and what you are thinking)

Each of the methods described here develop the concepts of place value and number sense. Number sense is fostered by presenting visual images, alongside the corresponding symbols, showing how numbers and operations are inter-related, for example 7 as $5 + 2$ and 10 as 2×5.

This is also the case for the number bonds for 10, for example, 10 can be 'seen' as $2 + 8$ or $6 + 4$ and so on. Place value is again covered with 100 as $20 + 80$ and $60 + 40$ and 1 as $0.2 + 0.8$ and $0.6 + 0.4$.

The comparison of adding or subtracting 9 via 10 is also an exercise in estimation aided by asking if the estimate is 'bigger or smaller?' Another good self-question for this task is, 'If what I subtract, 9, is smaller than 10, then will my answer be smaller or bigger?'

Things to do and practise

By practising these links, learners should be taken away from a dependence on counting in ones and taken towards more effective and efficient ways of accessing facts that they cannot retrieve from memory. Practice could include questions such as, 'How many ways can you derive the answer to 7 + 6?' Practise estimates of answers, for example +10 and +9 or estimating 6 + 7 by using 6 + 6 or 7 + 7. Use objects to enhance memory for set patterns.

Chapter 10

Addition and Subtraction

As the topics and strands of maths develop, learners should move further and further away from counting in ones. The 'basic facts' or 'number bonds' are part of that process. The previous chapter looked at how these facts could be retrieved by methods that supported memory and sense of number. In this chapter the processes of addition and subtraction are extended to all numbers. Whilst using finger counting to work out 6 + 8 can be effective, it can be inefficient and prone to error, but using a similar strategy is not going to be feasible for examples such as 364 + 877 or 2009 − 743. Even if the counting strategy is used for the steps in a procedure, it will slow the procedure down, thus putting more demand on working memory and leading to errors.

The strategies that were explained in the last chapter use chunks, for example 7 is chunked as 5 + 2 rather than seven ones. As with all the themes in this book, this idea will be developed and used as the maths develops. The principle is that using familiar, automatic chunks reduces the load on working memory.

Vocabulary and language

The vocabulary and the language used when addition and subtraction are put into word problems would require a chapter of its own (Chinn 2017a). In this chapter addition and subtraction are only presented as number problems. Later, in Chapter 20, we will look at word problems built around all four operations.

The vocabulary used in this chapter will centre on the key concepts, that is, place value and crossing the places (another example of an alternate phrase, used here, is 'bridging the tens'). A variety of words have been used at different times in the history of maths in schools for the process of 'trading' 10 ones for 1 ten and vice-versa, as explained in the previous chapter. For example, changing 1 ten to 10 ones has been called 'decomposition' and 're-grouping' and 'renaming'. There was also a variation on this which was called 'borrow and pay-back'. Teachers should make clear which vocabulary they are going to use and model it with materials and/or visual images so that the learner understands. So, if the teacher says, 'I am going to decompose', it is best if the learner knows that this refers to a specific procedure in maths. It is worth bearing in mind that a previous teacher may have preferred, for example, 'rename'. The pupil needs to know that the teacher is referring to the same procedure, but is using a different word.

Addition is what is known as 'commutative'. This means that it does not matter in which order you add numbers, the total will be the same, for example, $721 + 52 = 52 + 721 = 773$.

This is not true for subtraction, for example $600 - 10$ does not give the same answer as $10 - 600$.

Different word order can lead to confusion. For example, '70 take away 50' presents the 70 and 50 in the order for the symbols used in the calculation, $70 - 50$. But 'Take 50 away from 70' does not.

Images, symbols and concepts

The key prerequisite concepts are place value and trading. As ever, maths is developmental. The role of zero may also require specific attention and instruction. As with any topic in maths, if the prerequisite concepts are not understood, then the grasp on the new topic may well be insecure.

Since trading and place value are key concepts it is likely that base 10 blocks and coins will create effective kinaesthetic and visual images.

It is useful to remember that addition and subtraction are complementary operations. Adding is about putting numbers together. Subtraction is about splitting up numbers.

$$5 + 2 = 7 \qquad 7 - 2 = 5$$

Algebra often expresses ideas succinctly, and it generalises and shows patterns, which makes it such a shame that people shy away from it. In this example:

Addition is: $A + B = C$ e.g. $25 + 63 = 88$

Subtraction is: $C - B = A$ e.g. $88 - 63 = 25$

The relevance of the topic/concept to developing maths skills

Adding and subtracting are important skills for life, particularly for money (though maybe less so these days with touch cards). They are also prerequisite skills for multiplication and division. Another maths example is calculating a mean or average which also requires accurate addition skills.

THE TASK

Written procedures for adding and subtracting usually follow the sequence of place value, that is, ones, tens, hundreds, thousands and onwards. The process moves from right to left on the page, small place values to large place values. This is opposite to our normal writing and reading direction. Early maths so often appears to be inconsistent.

The first examples shown below do not require any bridging (or crossing) of place values. The procedures can be modelled with base 10 blocks, but only symbols are used here.

7432
+2516 Ones: $2 + 6 = 8$ Tens: $3 + 1 = 4$ Hundreds: $4 + 5 = 9$ Thousands: $7 + 2 = 9$
9948   (8)   (40)   (900)   (9000)

9948
-7432 Ones: $8 - 2 = 6$ Tens: $4 - 3 = 1$ Hundreds: $9 - 4 = 5$ Thousands: $9 - 7 = 2$
2516   (6)   (10)   (500)   (2000)

For the second group of examples, there is 'trading' from ones to tens for addition and from tens to ones for subtraction. The examples are modelled with images of base 10 blocks. Apart from the 'trading' these examples are the same as the first examples. The ones are added, then the tens are added.

57   **57**
+26   **+26**   First add the ones: $7 + 6 = 13$
                 $7 + 6 =$ 13
           $50 + 20 =$ **+70**   Then add the tens: $50 + 20 = 70$
                      83   Now add the two sub-additions: $70 + 13 = 83$

With base 10 blocks:

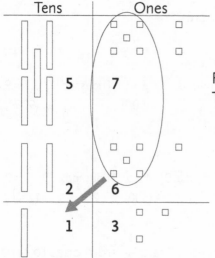

Tens | Ones

5   7

First add the ones: 7 + 6 = 13
Trade ten one cubes for a ten block

2   6

1   3

Now add the tens, that is 5 tens + 2 tens plus the 'traded' ten, 5 + 2 + 1 = 8 tens.

The final answer is 83.

Now look at subtraction. It is about reversing the process. (Note that some learners find reversing a process quite difficult, so the steps need to be presented comprehensively and clearly.) The 'trading' is illustrated with base 10 blocks.

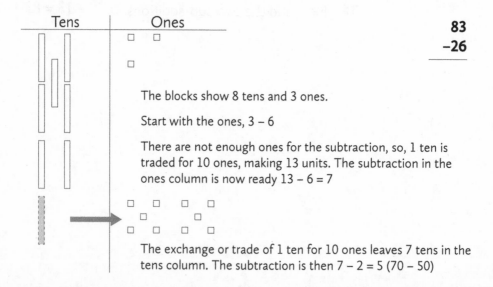

Tens | Ones

83
−26

The blocks show 8 tens and 3 ones.

Start with the ones, 3 − 6

There are not enough ones for the subtraction, so, 1 ten is traded for 10 ones, making 13 units. The subtraction in the ones column is now ready 13 − 6 = 7

The exchange or trade of 1 ten for 10 ones leaves 7 tens in the tens column. The subtraction is then 7 − 2 = 5 (70 − 50)

The answer is 57, which, of course, tallies with the numbers used in the corresponding addition problem.

Subtracting when zero is involved

The subtraction problems that often cause most difficulties are those that involve a zero, for example 304 – 67. However, the logic remains the same...there will have to be some trading to create more ones for the subtraction in the ones column. The confusion arises because there are no tens in the tens column for use for trading; trading will need to start at the first available place, in this case, the hundreds column.

If this is understood as the objective, to get some ones into the ones column, then the logic is to use the knowledge of the place value system to do this.

The first practice could be confined to trading to get more ones:

For 201, trading makes it 1 hundred plus 9 tens, plus 11 ones = 100 + 90 + 11

Hundreds	Tens	Ones

201 is now 1 hundred and 10 tens and one

Now a trade of 1 ten for 10 ones creates more ones

The 2 hundreds and 1 one has become 1 hundred, 9 tens and 11 ones and the subtraction can begin:

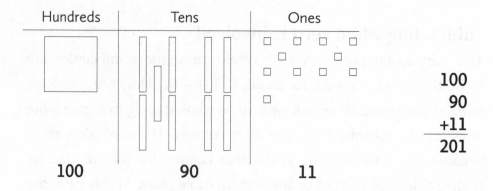

Hundreds	Tens	Ones

			100
-----	-----	-----	90
100	90	11	+11
			201

This procedure might be written without the 'scaffolding'/support of place value columns as:

$$\begin{array}{ccc} & 9 & 11 \\ 1 & \cancel{10} & \\ \cancel{2} & 0 & 1 \end{array}$$

Or, perhaps more clearly by using two extra lines for the two trading steps:

H	T	O	
2	0	1	
1	10	1	(trade 1 hundred for 10 tens)
1	9	11	(trade 1 ten for 10 ones)

The skill is to take a number and change the way it is made up, breaking it into parts without changing its value.

This skill can be used for trading in additions and subtractions, but remember it was also used for basic facts such as 7 + 7, which can be changed to 5 + 2 + 5 + 2 = 5 + 5 + 2 + 2 = 10 + 4 = 14.

Maths can progress by taking an idea or skill and extending it to new areas and problems. This is much better for memory and understanding than seeing each extension of an idea as something completely new, instead of a development of previous understanding.

Meta-cognition (thinking about how and what you are thinking)

As number sense develops, students can start to estimate answers before starting to compute and appraise answers after computation. The level of sophistication used for this can be refined as confidence grows. For example, for 57 + 26, the first attempt could be 50 + 20 = 70. The next attempt could be to consider the ones, which will add to make more than 10 (since both are more than 5), taking the estimate to 80.

Each problem should be overviewed to see if there are alternative and better ways to tackle it. As is stated above, it can be very helpful to understand how ideas develop and inter-relate: to know *why* you can use a method or a formula to solve a problem.

An alternative method for 57 + 26 could be 55 + 25 + 2 + 1 = 80 + 3 = 83.

Place value is very much a part of subtraction and addition, in particular knowing how to exchange/trade/regroup/rename numbers, as in seeing 673 as 500 + 160 + 13 or seeing 507 as 490 + 17. Students need to be able to 'see' numbers in different forms and combinations.

A pragmatic example of meta-cognition is the strategy of 'casting out tens'. One of the goals I have for a learner is that they become less of an impulsive problem solver and more of a reflective problem solver. I want them to overview and reflect on a problem before they attempt the solution. I want them to think about how they will think about the problem. 'Casting out tens' can be used an early experience of this strategy.

Here is an example. Add the numbers:

25   47   81   16   33   54   82   79   68

The addition could be done sequentially, adding the ones digits in the order they are given, then doing the same for the tens digits. (This could also be considered as an inchworm strategy.) This requires several addition steps, each of which may be a challenge (and a potential source of error) if the pupil is not secure in the retrieval of number facts.

If the numbers are overviewed, then it is usually possible to find number combinations (number bonds) for 10, for example:

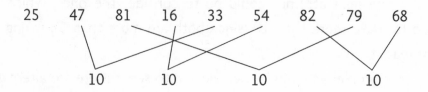

Only the 5 (from 25) has not been paired. The total for the ones is 40 + 5 = **45**.

Now look at the tens digits (with the 45 from the ones total included) and find the number combinations for 100.

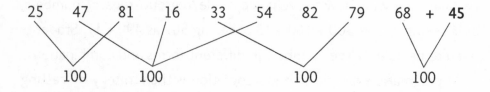

Only the 80 (from 82) has not been combined. The total for the tens is 400 + 80 = 480, making the total 485.

The cognitive strategy is to look at the numbers before starting to add them, to see if there is another way to add, using facts in an efficient and user-friendly way. In a sense this strategy is a variation on the chunking strategy.

A very basic estimation of the total can be obtained with an overview of the numbers. There are 9 two-digit numbers with a spread of values (not all near 100, not all near 10), so take an average number value of 50 and multiply it by 9 giving an estimate of 450. This can prevent 'big' errors such as the place value error, 45 + 44 = 89 (instead of 45 + 440).

Things to do and practise

Practise trading, crossing tens and hundreds with materials such as base 10 blocks or coins, but also with symbols (the digits and numbers). This practising need not involve actual adding or subtracting; just rename numbers, for example 72 as 60 + 12 (as the French language does anyway!).

Chapter 11

Basic Facts for Multiplication and Division

The times table facts are probably a child's first experience of persistent failure. Luckily this is not true for every child, but I suspect that it is a very significant percentage, particularly among those who are dyslexic. It should be noted that even when children do commit this body of facts to memory, it does not guarantee that they will understand the principles that underlie them, nor that they will remember them when they are older, when there is less practising and less recall.

It is also likely to be a child's first experience of the consequences of a maths belief, implicitly inferred or explicitly stated. That belief is that children, all children, can and should learn the times tables. A secondary belief is that maths will be very difficult if these facts are not retrievable, quickly, from memory.

These somewhat simplistic beliefs are not correct for every child and neither are they reasonable. The basis for my counter-beliefs is that there is an alternative and it is a mathematical alternative with cognitive benefits. And they are attainable. But the belief in the efficacy of 'learning by heart' is a very entrenched belief, often coupled with a sense of superiority.

For many people, the problematic facts lie in the bottom right-hand corner of the multiplication square. It seems like a small problem... unless you can't do it.

×	0	1	2	3	4	5	6	7	8	9	10
0											
1											
2											
3											
4											
5											
6											
7											
8											
9											
10											

Vocabulary and language

Once again, the vocabulary is not helpful in communicating the concept and once again there is no consistency. Let's start with, 'What is multiplication?' and the standard reply, 'Repeated addition'. Adding a column of different numbers could be interpreted as 'repeated addition'. In this specific case, multiplication, it means, 'Repeated addition of the same number'.

An example would be $6 + 6 + 6 + 6 + 6 + 6 + 6 = 7 \times 6$.

Then there is a range of vocabulary to infer multiplication, including, 'times', 'lots of', 'product' and nothing at all, as in 'What are six sevens?' That is a question where you need to know the maths (lack of) language code.

If the definition of multiplication involves 'repeated addition' then it would follow that the inverse operation, division, should be 'repeated subtraction of the same number'. The two definitions emphasise the link between the two operations.

There is a smaller range of vocabulary for division, including 'share' and 'How many...in...?', 'What is 25 over 5?', 'per' as in 'percentage... divided by 100' and nothing as in 3/5 or $\frac{3}{5}$

But there is, as with subtraction, an issue with the order of words. For example, 460 divided by 5 gives the numbers and the operation word in the correct order for keying into a calculator or for writing in symbols, $460 \div 5$.

The order of the wording for 'How many tens in 500?' does not work for a calculator, but it might help for the 'bus stop' presentation:

$$10 \overline{)500}$$

Images, symbols and concepts

The symbols used to infer multiplication and subtraction are more varied than the solitary + and − used for addition and subtraction. Again, consistency is not there to reassure the learner.

For multiplication we can use:

- × as in 5×7

- indices as in 8^2 which means 8×8

- brackets as in $5(4 + 3)$ which means $5 \times 4 + 5 \times 3$

- nothing at all, as in algebra, where ab means $a \times b$.

For division we can use:

- $\div$ as in $10 \div 2$

- the 'bus stop' layout for the division procedure $2\overline{)10}$

- a negative index as in 25^{-2}

- a stroke as in $5/10$

- a line with one number above another number as in $\dfrac{5}{7}$

A reminder: all four operations are interlinked, a concept that can be used constructively to provide alternative ways to solve problems.

The relevance of the topic/concept to developing maths skills

If the definition of multiplication is taken as repeated addition of the same number then aspects of algebra follow, for example:

$$2 + 2 + 2 + 2 = 4 \times 2$$
$$5 + 5 + 5 + 5 = 4 \times 5$$
$$8 + 8 + 8 + 8 = 4 \times 8$$
$$a + a + a + a = 4 \times a = 4a$$

If these repeated additions are collected into chunks, then the process of 'long' multiplication follows, a process that depends on partial products, for example:

$$7 + 7 + 7 + 7 + 7 + 7 + 7 + 7 + 7 + 7 + 7 + 7 = 10 \times 7 + 2 \times 7 = (10 + 2) \times 7$$

The links between multiplication and division are relevant in many areas of maths (see also the next chapter). For example, it helps to be able to relate these three equations and to understand their relationship:

$$6 \times 3 = 18$$
$$6 = 18 \div 3 \qquad \text{or} \quad \frac{18}{3}$$
$$3 = 18 \div 6 \qquad \text{or} \quad \frac{18}{6}$$

This is relevant to many equations/formulas such as:

$$\text{Distance} = \text{Speed} \times \text{Time} \qquad D = S \times T$$

or $\quad$ Speed $= \dfrac{\text{Distance}}{\text{Time}}$

or $\quad$ Time $= \dfrac{\text{Distance}}{\text{Speed}}$

Such three component equations are sometimes presented in a triangle as an aide-memoire for the inter-relationships. It's good to be able to understand why.

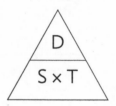

(There is also a clue in the units used for speed 'miles per hour' or 'kilometres per hour'. Miles and kilometres are for distance and hour is for time, so speed is equal to distance per time, and 'per' means divide.)

Meta-cognition (thinking about how and what you are thinking)

Remembering the basic multiplication and division facts is beneficial, but knowing how they inter-relate – how facts can be combined to find new facts (often via partial products) – means that the benefits will be far greater.

In the equation above, $S = D \times T$, it may help to relate it to a basic fact which is known comfortably and accurately, such as $2 \times 5 = 10$. The two other forms then follow and verify themselves:

$$5 = \frac{10}{2} \quad \text{and} \quad 2 = \frac{10}{5}$$

Children need to be taught how to understand the concepts of multiplication and division, how to think around the ways they can be used in other applications, such as percentages, area, algebra and fractions. They need to realise that in an equation like $xy = \text{constant}$, then as x gets bigger, y gets smaller. This can lead to understanding sequences such as:

$$12 \div 12 = 1$$
$$12 \div 6 = 2$$
$$12 \div 3 = 4$$
$$12 \div 2 = 6$$
$$12 \div 1 = 12$$
$$12 \div \tfrac{1}{2} = 24$$

and thus, to the realisation that, in certain situations, division can make the answer bigger (than the divided number).

Although the culture and beliefs around maths seem to be that basic facts are always retrieved in one step, there is a strong case for arguing that two steps are a very viable and mathematically alternative way of thinking about some of these 'facts'. Meta-cognition comes from knowing how partial products work for multiplication and for division. This knowledge leads us to alternative ways to multiply and divide.

THE TASK

The task is to be able to access all the basic times and division facts, by recall or by strategy, as swiftly as possible (without raising anxiety).

One possibility is to use mnemonics. I confess that I am not a great fan of the extensive use of mnemonics. The odd one here and there, like 'Richard Of York Gave Battle In Vain' for the colours of the rainbow 'Red, Orange, Yellow, Green, Indigo, Violet' is great, but to create a whole book of them dedicated to mnemonics for times table facts is making *War and Peace* out of a nursery rhyme. However, if it works, it works. But remember that recall on its own isn't cognition.

A powerful rote-learning strategy is the self-voice echo strategy of Dr Colin Lane, where the facts or information to be learned are recorded, *in the learner's own voice* on a PC, with a matching visual on the screen. That fact is then repeated back time and again (well, it is rote learning), preferably through headphones. My own research into this (Lane and Chinn 1986) showed that when it works, it works dramatically and with long-lasting retention. But it doesn't work for everyone, which is a valuable lesson for anyone who thinks they may have found 'the' cure for learning difficulties.

A method based on meta-cognition relates back to some early maths concepts.

First: let's consider the definition and understanding of what this collection of facts is:

It is a collection of repeated additions, relating to the vocabulary, 'lots of'. For example

6 × 8 is	8 + 8 + 8 + 8 + 8 + 8	6 lots of 8	and
7 × 7 is	7 + 7 + 7 + 7 + 7 + 7 + 7	7 lots of 7	

Second: you can cluster these additions into chunks rather than add on one number at a time. The 'chunks' that help are likely to be the ones using the 'easy' numbers: 1, 2, 5 and 10. In terms of cognitive style, this will appeal more to grasshopper than inchworms.

The chunks, for example, for 6 × 8 are 5 × 8 and 1 × 8 which are 40 and 8. These are 'partial products'. (A product is the outcome of a multiplication. Partial products can be combined to make the complete product.) So, then the 40 and the 8 can be added to make 48, the product for 6 × 8.

$$\overbrace{8 + 8 + 8 + 8 + 8} + 8$$

For 7 × 7 the process can also be done as two partial products:

$$\overbrace{7 + 7 + 7 + 7 + 7} + \overbrace{7 + 7}$$

$$5 \times 7 = 35 \qquad 2 \times 7 = 14 \qquad 35 + 14 = 49$$

Partial products can be combined by adding, or extended by multiplying, for example, 4 × 7 can be accessed via 2 lots of 2 × 7:

$$4 \times 7 = 2 \times 7 \times 2 = 2 \times 14 = 28$$

This strategy re-defines what makes a basic fact 'basic'. The **key** basic facts are the minimum number of facts that you need to work out other facts efficiently. They are the 1x, 2x, 5x and 10x facts for a number. For example, for the 8 times table, the core basic facts are:

$$1 \times 8 = 8$$
$$2 \times 8 = 16$$
$$5 \times 8 = 40$$
$$10 \times 8 = 80$$

These four partial products can be combined to access all the other 8x table facts, and some extra facts, too.

$1 \times 8 = 8$

$2 \times 8 = 16$

$3 \times 8 = 24$ $3 \times 8 = 2 \times 8 + 1 \times 8 = 16 + 8 = 24$

$4 \times 8 = 32$ $4 \times 8 = 2 \times 8 + 2 \times 8$ OR $2 \times (2 \times 8) = 16 + 16 = 32$

$5 \times 8 = 40$

$6 \times 8 = 48$ $6 \times 8 = 5 \times 8 + 1 \times 8 = 40 + 8 = 48$

$7 \times 8 = 56$ $7 \times 8 = 5 \times 8 + 2 \times 8 = 40 + 16 = 56$

$8 \times 8 = 64$ $8 \times 8 = 2 \times 2 \times 2 \times 8 = 2(2 \times 16) = 2 \times 32 = 64$

$9 \times 8 = 72$ $9 \times 8 = 10 \times 8 - 1 \times 8 = 80 - 8 = 72$

$10 \times 8 = 80$

Extra facts:

$11 \times 8 = 88$ $11 \times 8 = 10 \times 8 + 1 \times 8 = 80 + 8 = 88$

$12 \times 8 = 96$ $12 \times 8 = 10 \times 8 + 2 \times 8 = 80 + 16 = 96$

$15 \times 8 = 120$ $15 \times 8 = 10 \times 8 + 5 \times 8 = 80 + 40 = 120$

$19 \times 8 = 152$ $19 \times 8 = 20 \times 8 - 1 \times 8 = 2 \times 10 \times 8 - 1 \times 8 = 160 - 8 = 152$

The principle that underpins this strategy is the principle that underpins 'long' multiplication.

Division facts are the complementary or reverse facts to the multiplication facts, for example, $6 \times 8 = 48$ is a multiplication fact. Two division facts are complementary, for example, $48 \div 6 = 8$ and $48 \div 8 = 6$. These two division facts could be written as $6 \times ? = 48$ and $8 \times ? = 48$, thus interlinking division and multiplication. If the multiplication facts are known, then the ability to visualise them in this form will give the division facts.

The answers to division questions and facts can be accessed from the key basic facts. Where multiplication is repeated addition of the same numbers, division is repeated subtraction of the same numbers. For example, to access $72 \div 8$, subtract partial products:

The two partial products that will be used in this example are:

$2 \times 8 = 16$ and $5 \times 8 = 40$

Start by subtracting 40 $(\mathbf{5} \times \mathbf{8})$ $72 - 40 = 32$

then 16 $(\mathbf{2} \times \mathbf{8})$ $32 - 16 = 16$

and 16 $(\mathbf{2} \times \mathbf{8})$ $16 - 16 = 0$

9 lots of 8 have been subtracted so $72 \div 8 = 9$

Partial products can be demonstrated with Cuisenaire rods. Take the examples, $9 \times 8 = 72$ and $72 \div 8 = 9$.

First, for $72 \div 8$ use 9 'eight rods'. (The area this creates represents the 72.)

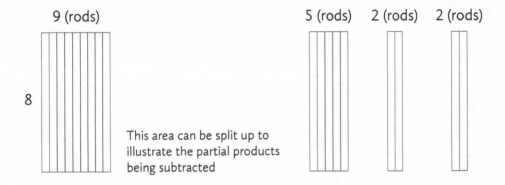

This image relates to the written presentation for division:

$$8\overline{)72}$$ with quotient 9

To demonstrate 9×8, the rods can be put together as three partial products, 5×8 and 2×8 and 2×8.

'5 lots of 8, plus 2 lots of 8 plus 2 lots of 8.'

Things to do and practise

Practise and learn the key basic facts described above. Practise combining them to make other facts.

Write the key facts on cards and play memory games with them, for example, after spreading a number of (8× or another number) cards face down on a table ask questions such as, 'Find two cards that can make 56.' (It will be a 5 × 8 card and a 2 × 8 card.)

Use the rods to demonstrate how areas are constructed and split up (de-constructed) using partial products.

Chapter 12

Multiplying and Dividing by 10, 100 and 1000 (Part 1)

The National Numeracy Strategy (DFES 2001) expected that 9-year-old pupils could: 'Multiply and divide any positive integer up to 10 000 by 10 or 100 and understand the effect'. My research for my standardised test (Chinn 2017b) suggests that this is not the case for more than a third of 15-year-old students in the UK and over a half of 13- and 10-year-olds. The percentages are for correct answers:

$$10\overline{)6030}$$ 10 years, 44.5%   13 years, 48.7%   15 years, 62.3%

Vocabulary and language

Basic vocabulary, such as '10 times bigger' or 'a hundred times smaller' may not be truly understood, particularly with area or volume.

The vocabulary will include 'indices' and 'the power of' which are likely to be unfamiliar to many learners. 'The power of' has the disadvantage of using an everyday word in a very specific maths context.

Prefixes

Knowing what the prefixes used in measurement mean is key information.

μ	micro	means one millionth	1/1 000 000	(÷ 1 000 000)	**very small**
m	milli	means one thousandth	1/1000	(÷ 1000)	
c	centi	means one hundredth	1/100	(÷ 100)	
k	kilo	means one thousand	1000	(× 1000)	
M	mega	means one million	1 000 000	(× 1 000 000)	**very big**

The world of computers uses prefixes, including some for huge numbers; for example a gigabyte is a billion bytes, 1 000 000 000.

A yottabyte is:

1 000 000 000 000 000 000 000 000

Once at a thousand, the prefixes are for multiples of 1000, for example: a thousand thousands, a million, is Mega and a thousand millions, a billion, is Giga.

(Note how the zeros are clustered in groups of three. Three items are within the subitising capacity of many people, so clusters of three make the communication of these large numbers more effective.)

Images, symbols and concepts

Mathematicians often look for ways to represent numbers and ideas about numbers in as succinct a way as they can devise. The number of zeros written after the 1 for the yottabyte is 24, which takes a while to write. The symbol code used to replace the writing of all those zeros is the 'index', so 1 000 000 000 000 000 000 000 000 becomes 10^{24} where 24 is the index.

The other vocabulary for this is '10 to the power of 24', which I quite like as the word 'power' suggests to me that something powerful is going on.

The logic behind powers can be seen in the sequence (or pattern) below:

$1 = 10^0$ (one)
$10 = 10^1$ (ten)
$100 = 10 \times 10 = 10^2$ (hundred)
$1000 = 10 \times 10 \times 10 = 10^3$ (thousand)
$10\,000 = 10 \times 10 \times 10 \times 10 = 10^4$ (ten thousand)
$100\,000 = 10 \times 10 \times 10 \times 10 \times 10 = 10^5$ (hundred thousand)
$1\,000\,000 = 10 \times 10 \times 10 \times 10 \times 10 \times 10 = 10^6$ (million)

The logic extends to dividing by 10 and powers of 10. The code is modified by including a minus sign in front of the index, for example, 10^{-2} means 'divide by 100' or 1/100 and 10^{-6} means divide by one million or 1/1 000 000.

The sequence is:

$$10^6 \quad 10^5 \quad 10^4 \quad 10^3 \quad 10^2 \quad 10^1 \quad 10^0 \quad 10^{-1} \quad 10^{-2} \quad 10^{-3} \quad 10^{-4} \quad 10^{-5} \quad 10^{-6}$$

Note the index in the middle is 0. 10^0 is 1.

Recognising patterns makes understanding and remembering more effective.

These tasks are very much about place value. They are often not well understood. Children rely on mnemonics, like '100 has 2 zeros so when you multiply a number by 100 you add 2 zeros to the number', for example $267 \times 100 = 26700$. If I wanted to interpret the mnemonic literally, and many students will react that way, then I might do:

```
  267
+ 00
-----
  267
```

This 'adding zeros' will not work with decimal numbers, for example 14.6 × 100 is *not*14.600. Instead, use the place value of a digit from the number, say 4 ones. When multiplied by 100 it becomes 4 hundreds. The other digits follow to give 1460.

It is also worth checking whether the pupil understands and can visualise what '10 times bigger' or 'a thousand times bigger' actually means.

The images for demonstrating '10 times bigger' or '10 times smaller' could be the base 10 blocks. For these to be effective, the pupil needs to be able to perceive value in objects that are 3D and in 3D objects that are drawn as 2D shapes.

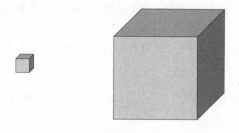

For example, if 1 is represented by a cube that has sides of 1cm, then a cube with sides of 10cm will represent 1000 and a cube with sides of 100cm (1m) will represent 1 000 000. This is using volume. Volume could be used, with containers for 1millilitre, 10ml, 100ml and 1000ml (one litre), but the pupil needs to be able to appreciate the way volume represents quantity.

A linear image of the proportions involved for × or ÷ 10, 100, 1000 could be a metre rule, marked in decimetres, centimetres and millimetres.

Money can be used, but this relies on a clear understanding that a £1 coin represents a value that is 100 times bigger than a 1 pence coin, and that a £10 note represents 1000 one pence coins. Coins and notes are not proportional to the quantities they represent, and, just to confuse some learners, we usually write pence as decimals as in £23.56.

Manipulatives/materials are important, but they often have different characteristics and different relevance to individual pupils *and always* they must be directly and clearly linked to the relevant symbols.

The key concept here is, once again, place value and that involves symbols and symbols in sequences.

The relevance of the topic/concept to developing maths skills

Harder problems for multiplication and division, sometimes known as 'long' multiplication and 'long' division, require an understanding of and a facility with multiplying and dividing by 10, 100, 1000 and onwards to other powers of 10.

Measurement and the units used for measurement (for example, 1 metre, 1 centimetre is 1/100 of a metre, 1 millimetre is 1/1000 of a metre) also require an understanding of these skills and concepts.

Using 10, 100, 1000 and other powers of 10 are key to estimation.

An understanding of place value will also be key to rounding (up and down).

Being able to divide and multiply by 100 is required for percentages.

Decimals also require this knowledge and an understanding of its impact on place values.

THE TASK

The task is to be able to multiply and divide numbers by 10 and powers of 10 and to understand what happens, and why, to the numbers being multiplied or divided.

A non-decimal place value columns diagram is shown below to remind the pupils what the places for each digit in a number mean in terms of the value it represents.

Thousands	Hundreds	Tens	Ones
7	5	8	3
7000	500	80	3

(One aspect of the elegance of the Hindu-Arabic number system is that you do not have to write the value of each digit. If this was done then seven thousand, five hundred and eighty-three would become rather a lot of digits: 7000 500 80 3.)

When a number is multiplied by 10, each digit in the number moves one place (to the left) to now represent a quantity that is 10 times bigger. For example, $486 \times 10 = 4860$:

Thousands	Hundreds	Tens	Ones
	4	8	6
4	8	6	0

The 4 (400) has become 4000.
The 8 (80) has become 800.
The 6   (6) has become 60.

Each digit has moved one place up in value. The answer 4860 is 10 times bigger than 486.

The digits have not changed their sequence, but they have changed their place value. If the 6 were to be a focus, then 6×10 becomes 60, the 6 moves to the tens place and all the other digits move one place value to keep the sequence. The 0 in the ones column maintains the other digits in their correct place value column.

Another example, 3185 × 10 = 31850:

Ten thousands	Thousands	Hundreds	Tens	Ones
	3	1	8	5
3	1	8	5	0

Again, the sequence of digits is the same, and they follow the ones digit (5) which is now a tens digit, because 5 × 10 = 50.

The same principle applies for multiplying by 100, for example 179 × 100 = 17900:

Ten thousands	Thousands	Hundreds	Tens	Ones
		1	7	9
1	7	9	0	0

Once more the sequence of digits remains the same, but each digit has moved 2 places. A focus on the ones digit, 9, shows that it is now in the hundreds place since 9 × 100 = 900. The other digits follow the move and the zero holds their places.

The relationship between multiplication and division is that one is the reverse of the other, so it should be predictable that the division by 10, 100 and other powers of 10 will be the opposite to the multiplication. So, for the example directly above, the complementary division will be 17900 ÷ 100:

Ten thousands	Thousands	Hundreds	Tens	Ones
1	7	9	0	0
		1	7	9

The 9 digit in the hundreds place has become a 9 digit in the ones place (900 ÷ 100 = 9).

The other digits move to the right in the same sequence.

Meta-cognition (thinking about how and what you are thinking)

These procedures for multiplying and dividing by powers of 10 should enhance the understanding of place value. The values of numbers multiplied or divided by powers of 10 can be compared, first by looking at how many digits and then comparing the values of the individual digits that make up the number.

This awareness should also enhance the ability to appraise answers. For example, in the data for my test for the item on column addition:

```
 37
 42
 73
+68
```

A common error was 40 (the digits in the ones column add to 20 and the digits in the tens column also add to make 20, so, erroneously, 20 + 20 = 40). This answer is simply not possible at even the most superficial of appraisals! A cognitive approach to appraising an approximate answer is to look at the 4 numbers, estimate that each could be 50, then 4 × 50 = 200. The answer must have 3 digits, even if only 73 and 68 are added.

Multiplying and dividing by 10 and powers of 10 is used in measurement.

It is a useful skill for estimations when converting money on trips abroad.

It will help when developing an understanding of percentages.

Things to do and practise

Practise writing some problems for ×10, ×100, ×1000 and looking at the sequence of digits.

Do some multiplication and division problems mentally.

Convert some measurements, for example, 'How many metres in 5 kilometres?' or 'How many kilograms is 3000 grams?

Rounding up and down

Rounding a number up or down to the nearest ten, or hundred or thousand and so on is a skill that draws on knowledge of place value and a sense of number size. There is also one convention to deal with the half-way numbers: 5, 50, 500 and so on. 5 is always rounded up.

I was introduced to a version of this diagram by a Filipino teacher. I have modified it from a vertical orientation to a horizontal image.

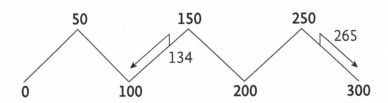

The idea is that any number will go down the slope to the rounded value at the bottom of the slope. The convention tells us to take 5, 50, 500 and so on, and roll them to the bigger ten, hundred, thousand and so on.

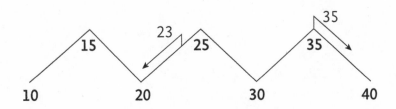

In this 10 to 40 diagram, the 23 rolls to 20 and the 35 rolls to 40. In the 0 to 300 diagram the 134 rolls back to 100 and the 265 rolls forward to 300.

Chapter 13

Multiplication and Division

Once the problem of the basic facts has been addressed, the next step is to be able to compute longer/harder problems for multiplication and division. The data collected to create the norm-referenced maths test in my book on diagnosing maths difficulties (Chinn 2017b) revealed low levels of performance in these tasks. For example, the percentages from this large (1783) sample of UK school children who achieved the *correct* answers for the questions were very low:

For $9 \overline{)927}$

10 years, 14.5%   13 years, 31.4%   15 years, 46.8%

For   541
       ×203

10 years, 14.1%   13 years, 15.2%   15 years, 38.2%

Poor abilities with such questions obviously stretch beyond the special needs population. *This could suggest that methods that are introduced for pupils with specific learning difficulties will help many more children as well.*

An example of the developmental nature of maths is that the strategies used to extend the key basic facts to other basic facts were based on partial products and these are now used in long multiplication. This concept will be developed further in this chapter.

The four operations are interlinked, a concept that can be used constructively to provide alternative ways to solve problems. For example, it is possible to obtain an answer to a subtraction problem by adding on. For example, to compute 100 – 63, start with 63 and add 7 to make 70, then add 30 to make 100. 30 + 7 have been added, so the answer is 37.

It is possible to divide by thinking of multiplication. For example, $42 \div 7 = ?$ could be written in a different order as $? \times 7 = 42$, becoming, 'What do I multiply 7 by to get 42?', but to do this there must be an understanding of that link between multiplication and division. Another example of this link is that 'long' multiplication is carried out by adding together partial products and 'long' division is carried out by subtracting partial products.

Vocabulary and language

Multiplication, like addition, is commutative. That means that the order in which you multiply numbers does not change the final answer, for example:

$$6 \times 5 = 5 \times 6 \quad \text{or} \quad 7 \times 8 \times 9 = 9 \times 8 \times 7$$

This is not true for division, where the sequence of numbers and symbols affects the answer, for example:

$$30 \div 6 = 5 \quad \text{but} \quad 30 \div 5 = 6 \quad \text{and} \quad 30 \div 6 = 5$$

$30 \div 6$ can be stated in words as 'thirty divided by six' where the order of the words matches the symbols. It could also be stated as, 'How many sixes in thirty?' where the order of the numbers is now reversed. There may also be an interpretation issue. 'How many sixes in thirty?' gives no clue as to the process that might lead to an answer. The learner needs to know the mathematical meaning of the vocabulary.

One of the fascinating errors for division I have encountered is:

$$\begin{array}{r} 01 \\ 5\overline{\smash{\big)}35} \end{array} \qquad \begin{array}{r} 02 \\ 4\overline{\smash{\big)}28} \end{array}$$

A guess as to the method used is, 'How many fives in 3? There aren't any, so 0. How many fives in 5? There's 1.' And 'How many fours in 2? There aren't any, so 0. How many fours in 8? 2.' Many of the errors encountered in the standardising data were probably down to part remembered procedures or mis-applications.

Images, symbols and concepts

There are some concepts and skills that are prerequisites for these tasks and this might be one reason for their apparent difficulty. The prerequisites have been forgotten. When a maths procedure becomes more complex and demands more steps, it obviously becomes more likely to create failure. If the learner is relying entirely on memorising the steps without any understanding, then only perfect recall will lead to accuracy. Just one mistake in that recall is all it takes to fail.

The key concepts (and prerequisite skills) are place value and the ability to understand and carry out multiplication and division by powers of 10. The methods for multiplication inevitably require an ability to add and subtract accurately. An ability to access the key basic facts is required as is an ability to organise work on the page. For the organisation problem it may be beneficial to provide (appropriately sized) squared paper for some pupils. The use, and understanding, of partial products which was introduced for accessing some basic facts is also a prerequisite skill.

The visual image that fits these procedures and the concepts of multiplication and division is a rectangle (or square). It is area that illustrates the steps and the outcome. The area could be a simple drawing, or base 10 blocks or square counters or Cuisenaire rods.

The relevance of the topic/concept to developing maths skills

Multiplication and division are used widely in topics in maths. For example, the basic relationships of A × B = C and A = C ÷ B are used for topics such as:

- area = height × width

- sine = opposite ÷ hypotenuse

- force = mass × acceleration

- euros = pounds × exchange rate

- speed = distance ÷ time

- pounds = 2.2 × kilograms

- circumference = π × d.

THE TASK

As stated above, the analysis of the results used to standardise my 15-minute maths screener test suggests that multiplication and division skills are not well developed in the UK. One hypothesis is that the methods advocated are too reliant on recall and application of procedures which are not backed by understanding. Methods that make heavy demands on memory and do not offer a rationale for 'Why am I doing this?' do not suit the needs of many learners who experience learning difficulties. And we need to remember that meta-cognition is not the exclusive preserve of the more able and thus not patronise our learners.

Multiplication and division are essentially about partial products. If a multiplication or a division is perceived as being too difficult to compute in one step, then two or more steps can be used. The steps use partial products. For example, for 67 × 21:

Step 1   67 × 1 =   67   (67 is the first partial product)
Step 2:   67 × 20 = 1340   (1340 is the second partial product)
Step 3: Add the partial products 1407

Division follows the same pattern, but with subtraction, for example, 1407 ÷ 21

Step 1:   Subtract the partial product, **20** × 67   1407
                                                          −1340
                                                            67

Step 2:   Subtract the partial product, **1** × 67   − 67
                                                              0

Step 3:   Add **20 + 1** to give 21 as the answer

Meta-cognition (thinking about how and what you are thinking)

The concept used for basic facts is developed further for more complex multiplication and division problems. Adding and subtracting are also still present and so, if those skills are insecure, then multiplication and division will be insecure. Understanding is so important for securing the method in long-term memory. Learning how to think about the procedures and understand them, rather than relying solely on memory, is the meta-cognition. Being flexible and responsive to each different problem is also meta-cognition. The inter-relationship between multiplication and division enables students to move from the classic physics equation, $F = ma$, to $a = F/m$ and to think about the answer rather than simply writing down a number. For example, thinking about $a = F/m$ will tell the learner that a bigger mass (m) will experience a smaller acceleration (a) for a given force (F).

The link between multiplication and division could be visualised in the layout used for the traditional procedure for division. The sides of the frame

could be interpreted as two sides of a rectangle. So, for an area problem:

$$
\begin{array}{ccc}
71 & 71 & \text{width} \\
6\ \underline{426} & 6\ \boxed{426} & \text{height}\ \boxed{\text{area}}
\end{array}
$$

The three versions of the relationship are:

area   = width × height $426 = 71 \times 6$

width   = area ÷ height $71 = 426 \div 6$

height = area ÷ width $6 = 426 \div 71$

A further opportunity for meta-cognition is the breaking down and building up of numbers, for example, by using place value, 68 can be interpreted as 60 + 8, but by using key basic facts, 68 can, alternatively, be seen as 70 – 2. The first 'breakdown' results in two partial products, but the student will have to recall 6× and 8× multiplication facts. The second 'breakdown' results in more partial products, so 68 = 50 + 20 – 2, but all are the product of a key basic multiplication fact and more likely to be retrieved. The partial products can also be used as estimates and thus reduce the chance of 'big' errors. Examples of both strategies are given below:

716 × 68

Using place value to create partial products:

$$
\begin{array}{r}
716 \\
\times\ 68 \\
\hline
\end{array}
$$

```
 5728      (716 ×  8)
42960      (716 × 60)   This step is often done without the correct place value.
48688
```

Using key numbers to create partial products:

```
   716
 ×  68
 35800     (50 × 716)   This answer can be used as a very approximate estimate.
 14320     (20 × 716)
 50120     (70 × 716)   This answer can be used as a closer estimate.
```

Now we use $68 = 70 - 2$ and subtract 2×716

```
 50120     (70 × 716)
 -1432     ( 2 × 716)
 48688
```

There are more steps, but the method circumvents the barrier that occurs when 'harder' multiplication facts cannot be retrieved. This example also provides a very rough estimate ($50 \times 716 = 35800$) and a close estimate ($70 \times 716 = 50120$). The method uses the same concept of partial products as the 'traditional' method. It is about making a procedure accessible, rather than shorter. And for an extra check, some partial products are related by place value. In this example $2 \times 716 = 1432$ and $20 \times 716 = 14320$.

The same method can be applied to division. Division is likely to cause more difficulty and often will generate the 'no attempt' strategy. Consider the first step in the traditional method:

```
68 )‾4‾8‾6‾8‾8‾
```

'How many 68s in 486?' That is challenging for any student, but for those with a poor retrieval of basic facts, even more so.

The method used for multiplication, based on partial products from key basic facts, can be adapted to circumvent that 'getting started' barrier:

Step 1. Set up a table for the partial products of 68:

$$1 \times 68 = \quad\quad 68$$
$$10 \times 68 = \quad\quad 680$$
$$100 \times 68 = \quad 6800$$
$$2 \times 68 = \quad\quad 136$$
$$20 \times 68 = \quad\quad 1360$$
$$200 \times 68 = 13600$$
$$5 \times 68 = \quad\quad 340 \quad \text{(for a check, compare to } 10 \times 68 \text{...it should be half of 680)}$$
$$50 \times 68 = \quad 3400$$
$$500 \times 68 = 34000$$

(Setting up such tables is good revision for inter-relating partial products, such as 2×68 and 20×68 or 5×68 and 50×68.)

Step 2. Subtract the partial products of 68 from 48688:

48688	
− 34000	**500 × 68**
14688	
− 13600	**200 × 68**
1088	
− 680	**10 × 68**
408	
− 340	**5 × 68**
68	
− 68	**1 × 68**
716 × 68	

Again, the procedure is longer, but it may make an 'impossible' task into a possible one and there are built in checks by inter-relating the partial products.

Things to do and practise

Practise breaking down numbers by place value and by key numbers.

Practise doing long multiplications by both methods to investigate which works best for the learner and the particular example they are working on.

Practise multiplication involving powers of 10, for example × 5, × 50, × 500, × 5000. Compare the answers. Look for patterns.

Try pre-calculation estimates and post-calculation appraisals.

Looking at prerequisites and their impact on learners

As maths topics develop, they demand more prerequisite skills. For example, it is difficult to understand number bonds that create a two-digit answer without understanding place value. 'Long' multiplication, or any multiplication where partial products are used, requires the ability to add. Consequently, division requires an ability to subtract.

Multiplying and dividing by 10 and powers of 10 requires an understanding of place value. Later, multiplying by a fraction that is less than 1 challenges the belief, based on previous experience, that multiplying always results in a bigger answer.

Check if the prerequisite concepts and skills are there before embarking on teaching a new topic.

Intervention is often about knowing how far back to go to before you begin. That 'going back' will often be much further back than you might initially think. But 'going back' may also be brief, just enough to refresh memory.

Note: The 'grid method' was advocated for multiplication some years ago in England. The evidence from my standardisation data is that it is not working for too many pupils, but, see the next chapter for an illustration and explanation of the grid method. It could be another example of a blind application of a procedure resulting in errors.

Chapter 14

The Development of Multiplication

The Area Model

One of the themes in this book is that mathematics is developmental. The concepts develop, the facts develop and the skills develop. There are consequences. New topics often have prerequisite skills and concepts that need to be understood first. This leads to a compelling case for tracking back when planning an intervention: tracking back to find insecurities and tracking back to find the point where the learner is secure. The gaps in learning for students may often be in fundamental concepts. Place value is a frequent example of this, especially when zeros are involved.

The sequence of diagrams below acts as visual images of how the concept of multiplication develops. It is based on the visual presentation of multiplication as area. The diagrams represent base 10 blocks.

Stage 1.　　1 × 14. As 1 ten and 4 ones.

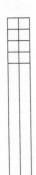

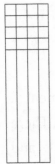

Stage 2.   2 × 14.   As 2 × 10   plus   2 × 4

= 20 + 8 = 28

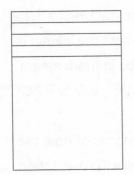

Stage 3.   4 × 14.   As 4 × 10   plus   4 × 4   OR

as 2 × 2 × 14 = 56

(The area is twice that of 2 × 14)

Stage 4.   10 × 14.   As 10 × 10 plus 10 × 4

= 100 + 40 = 140

Another illustration of place value and ×10.
The 4 ones become 4 tens and
the ten becomes 1 hundred.

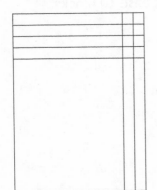

Stage 5.   12 × 14.   As 10 × 14 plus 2 × 14

= 140 + 28 = 168

This is an example of partial products.
This example relates back to strategies used
for basic facts, such as 7 × 6 = 5 × 6 + 2 × 6.
It relates onwards to 'bigger' multiplication
problems.

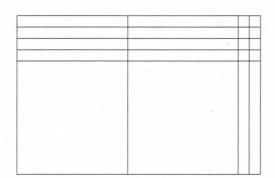

Stage 6.   22 × 14 = 308

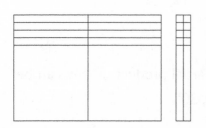

Stage 6a.   22 × 14
The image shows 20 × 14 plus 2 × 14.
20 × 14 is 10 × bigger than 2 × 14.
Also, it is 2 × bigger than 10 × 14.
Again, it is about place value and inter-relating numbers.

(The area model supports discussions about relative number values. These discussions should be encouraged.)

The next visual image shows how the 'grid method' works.

The multiplication 22 × 14 is broken down into 4 partial products as illustrated by 4 areas above.

The 4 areas are

$$
\begin{array}{rrcr}
20 \times & 10 & = & 200 \\
20 \times & 4 & = & 80 \\
2 \times & 10 & = & 20 \\
2 \times & 4 & = & 8 \\
\hline
& & & 308
\end{array}
$$

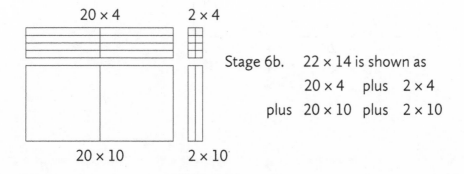

20 × 4   2 × 4

Stage 6b.   22 × 14 is shown as

20 × 4   plus   2 × 4

plus 20 × 10 plus   2 × 10

20 × 10   2 × 10

This leads to the grid method which uses digits only.

	20	2	
10	**200**	**20**	220
4	**80**	**8**	88
	280	28	308

The four numbers in bold are the four partial products. They can be added across or down to give the answer, 308.

Stage 7. Algebra

Algebra follows the same rules as used for numbers. Algebra often acts as a generalisation for all numbers. This step to the next stage may seem to some to be a challenging one, but it is closely linked to and developed from the stages that preceded it. Compare it to stages 6a and 6b above.

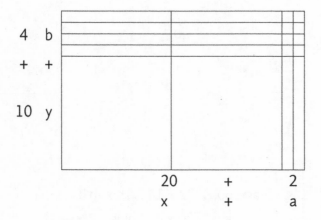

The illustration is the same as used for 22 × 14. The connection to algebra is that 22 is interpreted first as 20 + 2 and then in letters as x + a. 14 is interpreted first as 10 + 4 and then in letters as y + b. The area is (20 + 2) × (10 + 4) or (x + a)(y + b). Letters replace numbers.

$$(x + a)(y + b) = xy + bx + ay + ab$$

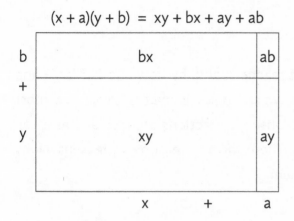

bx ab xy and ay and bx and ab are all partial products.

This visual is a good way of seeing how to work out (x + a)(y + b) = xy + bx + ay + ab) rather than as a mnemonic such as FOIL which tells to multiply the First (xy), the Outers (ab), the Inners (ay) and the Last (ab) letters.

Chapter 15

Fractions

In another of my surveys of teachers, and, by now another large and international sample, I ask which topics in maths cause the most problems for pupils. Not surprisingly, fractions are included as a top topic for causing difficulties. There will be a reason – or reasons – why this is such a universal problem.

Vocabulary and language

The fractions that are met most frequently, which are also the fractions that are used to introduce the topic, have unhelpful vocabulary. There are inconsistencies. The most frequently encountered fraction, a half, is a vocabulary exception to the naming rule for 1/5, 1/6, 1/7 onwards and in the way that the word 'twelve' gives no information about how to write the number, the word 'half' does not give any information about how to write the fraction.

'Third' and 'quarter' are also outside the pattern. The alternative for 'quarter', that is 'fourth', does fit the subsequent pattern. Another confusion may come from the use of all the words in the pattern fifth, sixth, seventh...to denote position in an order of things. (For example, 'I came fifth in that race.')

When multiplying by fractions, children meet the word 'of' which is used here to mean multiply. In everyday life, for example, when we say, 'Can I have three of those sweets, please?' 'of' does get interpreted as 'multiply'.

Language can be helpful in some examples of work with fractions. 'One fifth plus one fifth' is logically 'two fifths' and this helps when explaining how to add fractions that have the same name (or 'denominator'). One fifth plus one sixth is, linguistically, not possible to answer. This may support the argument that fractions sometimes have to be 're-named', the word we used for subtraction and addition, but with a different method attached to it for fractions.

Fractions challenge the consistency of previous experience of what happens when the operations multiply and divide are used. The outcomes of examples such as ¼ × 8 and 12 ÷ ½ are the opposite to the whole number examples previously encountered. Multiplication now gives a smaller answer and division a bigger answer. One of the ways these new outcomes can be explained is by using appropriate vocabulary and language. For division, the vocabulary that supports the concept is, 'How many halves in 12?' and 'How many halves make 12?' (an example of repeated addition), rather than 'What is 12 divided by a half?' For multiplication, 'What is a quarter of 8?' rather than, 'What is 8 times a quarter?' or 'What is 8 divided by 4?'

Images, symbols and concepts

Images used to teach fractions in schools often include pizzas. In fact, I wonder why a whole generation of children has not been put off eating pizza. Luckily most parents are unlikely to make this treat a test of skill with fractions: 'If Dave has 2/7 of the pizza, Lisa has 1/5 and Callum has 4/9, how much is left for Dad?'

Cuisenaire rods can be a useful manipulative for introducing and demonstrating fractions, but squares of plain paper, for folding or cutting up and thus dividing, can also provide a good demonstration of how fractions work. If a pedantic approach is taken to the topic, then pizzas (and cakes and apples) are not an acceptable image for fractions.

Fractions must be precise. Dividing a pizza in three pieces and for those pieces to be precisely equal is close to impossible, especially if there are lots of toppings. The same caution applies to half an apple.

Symbolic, abstract representation of information is often more of a problem for dyslexic and dyscalculic pupils so we need to use visual images or kinaesthetic experiences alongside the symbols. The kinaesthetic bit might make pizzas seem a good idea, but this is not mathematically accurate.

Fractions will challenge the learner's need for consistency and the security of knowing about multi-digit numbers and place value. There are other inconsistencies in work with fractions. For example, the question, 'What is one fifth plus one fifth?' has the logical (and correct) answer of 'Two fifths'. If this same problem is presented in symbols, the answer that is often given is two tenths, which is incorrect:

$$\frac{1}{5} + \frac{1}{5} = \frac{2}{10} = \text{wrong!}$$

There are some new rules to learn before fractions can be added. The logic of the + sign, to a non-mathematician, should be that it applies to both the top and the bottom numbers in the fraction. This is not the correct maths logic. However, seemingly inconsistently, the logic returns for multiplication where the × sign operates on top and bottom numbers:

$$\frac{2}{5} \times \frac{3}{5} = \frac{6}{25}$$

These inconsistencies are a serious barrier for many children. For a fraction item in my 15 minutes maths test (Chinn 2017b):

$$\frac{2}{5} + \frac{3}{8}$$

the percentage of *correct* answers for 13- and 14-year-old students were respectively 24.6 per cent and 39.1 per cent. It is sometimes very interesting (and often depressing) to know how the general population of students perform in maths.

The problem with the symbol code for fractions is that it hides a division sign. Ordinary two-digit numbers could be viewed as hiding a multiplication sign and an addition sign, for example:

$$47$$
$$4 \times 10 \quad + \quad 7 \times 1$$

Fractions hide the division sign with the line that separates the two numbers (top and bottom).

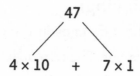

Of course, a division has a different outcome to a multiplication, which is why fractions obey different rules, one of which is that the fractions in the sequence

$$\frac{1}{2}, \frac{1}{3}, \frac{1}{4}, \frac{1}{5} \ldots$$

are getting smaller, but if the pupil focuses on the digits 1, 2, 3, 4, 5, previous experience has that sequence as getting bigger. Consistency is challenged unless the fractions are explained so that this misconception is addressed.

Adding fractions is more complicated than adding whole numbers or decimals, but there are some ideas in the next section.

The relevance of the topic/concept to developing maths skills

It is quite hard to make a strong case for the relevance of fractions in everyday life other than those in common usage: half, quarter, third and tenths. However, there is some transfer to the concept of proportion.

Meta-cognition (thinking about how and what you are thinking)

It is vital to think about the difference in the concept of a fraction to the concept of a whole number. The two digits or numbers involved in a fraction have different roles. The bottom number is about how many parts the whole has been divided into, for example for

$$\frac{2}{5}$$

the bottom digit tells us that the whole has been divided into 5 equal parts and the top digit tells us that we have 2 of them.

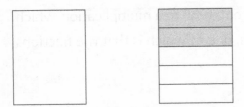

Another difference is in the idea of 'equivalent' fractions. A fraction can be expressed in more than one combination of numbers. The most common example is the half, 1/2, 1 out of 2. We meet a half as:

a half of an hour is 30 out of 60 minutes 30/60

half a £1 is 50 pence out of 100 pence, 50/100

half a kilometre is 500 metres out of 1000 metres, 500/1000

half a day is 12 hours out of 24 hours, 12/24

half a year is 6 months out of 12 months, 6/12.

Each of these fractions share a common characteristic. The top number is half of the bottom number, hence all these fractions are a half.

A simple, low cost manipulative for illustrating concepts and procedures with fractions is a sheet of paper. By folding the paper, fractions are created:

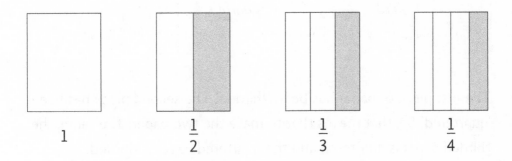

The images are simple (and not cluttered by pizza toppings). Discussions can introduce the vocabulary and concept of fractions, for example, 'This is 1 half. There are 2 halves made from the whole sheet of paper. There are 4 quarters. To make a quarter the half is halved again (divided by 2 again). 2 quarters can be added to make a half. A quarter and a third cannot be added (yet) as they are different sizes. They are not the same.'

The model (the paper sheet) has the main characteristic required of a material/manipulative, in that it directly relates to the concept, the symbols and the procedures, plus it is not a cluttered image.

The procedure for adding fractions that have different names, different denominators, is to rename them so that they do have the same name. In the case of 1/3 + 1/4 this requires both fractions to be renamed so that they do have the same name. It is about creating two equivalent fractions before the adding (or subtracting) can take place.

Equivalent means that the new fraction keeps the same value, but that the denominator and numerator are different to those in the original fraction, for example, 1/2 and 50/100.

Paper-folding can be used to model the procedure. The demonstration shows that, when both fractions have been changed to have the same name, it is possible to add them.

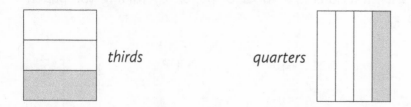

thirds   *quarters*

The first piece of paper has been 'thirded'. The second piece has been 'quartered'. So, that means that to make the two papers the same, the thirded paper is quartered and the quartered paper is thirded.

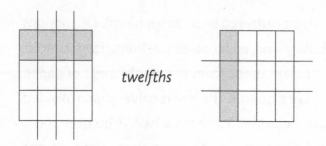

twelfths

Both whole papers are now showing 12/12. The 1/3 has become 4/12 and the ¼ has become 3/12. The two fractions now have the same name (twelfths) and can be added:

$$\frac{4}{12} + \frac{3}{12} = \frac{7}{12}$$

The explanation that should accompany this demonstration has to link the visual images to the symbols and steps in the standard procedure.

Empty number lines can be used to estimate answers, for example, 1/3 + 1/4:

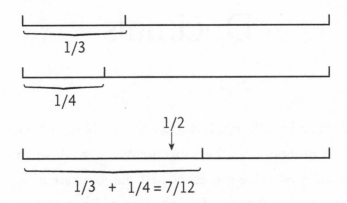

The answer is about a half, but it is more than a half. The estimate is used to prevent (or reveal) big mistakes. In this example, half is a useful comparison value. So, the estimate here would be 'about a half' or 'just more than a half'.

Things to do and practise

Practise renaming fractions to make equivalent fractions. Use the vocabulary alongside the symbols for mutual clarification. Perhaps use, for example, 'two fifths' alongside 'two out of five'.

Fold paper squares and relate the outcomes to the mathematical operations and symbols and write the fractions on the squares.

Use a number line (as below) for estimating answers. This skill is considered by a large USA research project to be a key indication that fractions are understood. Linking fractions to decimals can further support this skill.

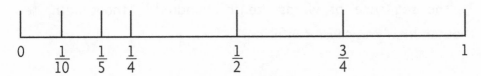

Chapter 16

Decimals

Our early experience of maths is with whole numbers, but as we grow up we meet part-numbers, numbers that are part of a whole, for example, a half. The main ways we represent part-numbers are as fractions, as decimals and as percentages. This chapter is about decimals and the way they can be understood as a development of place value.

The most common example of decimals that we meet is money, specifically pence. When we write a price, for example £16.85, the .85 is a decimal which is also, in this example, 85 pence. The 85 pence is a part (85/100) of a pound. It is not a whole pound.

In the USA, the equivalent of our pence is a cent. The word cent gives the clue as to its value. 'Cent' infers 100. There are 100 cents in a US dollar. The word 'pence' doesn't give us that clue, but there are 100 pence in a pound. This can also be understood as: 1 pence is one hundredth of a pound.

Vocabulary and language

Decimals are actually 'decimal fractions'. This means that they are fractions which have denominators (bottom numbers) that are specifically, 10, 100, 1000 and so on. So, decimals are about tenths, hundredths, thousandths and so on.

The sequence of words, 'tenth, hundredth, thousandth, ten thousandth...' can cause confusion.

There are three ways that this confusion can arise. First, the 'th' at the end of each of those words does not make much sound when you say the words. It can be quite tricky to hear the difference in sound between 'four hundred' and 'four hundredth'. The difference in value is that 'four hundred' is ten thousand times bigger than 'four hundredths'.

The other source of potential confusion is that the sequence, one, ten, hundred, thousand, ten thousand is a sequence that gets ten times *bigger* each step. The decimal sequence, tenth, hundredth, thousandth, ten thousandth is a sequence that gets ten times *smaller* each step.

The third source of potential confusion is that there is no 'oneth' (see below).

When we read decimals, such as 147.9, we say them as 'one hundred and forty-seven *point* nine'. The word 'point' warns the listener that the next digit to be spoken will represent a decimal. Maybe this is one of the contributors to the 'decimal point' (to give it its full name) being a focus of attention.

There has often been a strong focus in maths books on the 'decimal point'. This focus can be misleading conceptually.

Images, symbols and concepts

The reason that a focus on the decimal point has the potential for confusion is that the decimal point is not the centre of the symmetry between whole and part numbers. The focus is the ones. To understand the concept of decimals the focus of instruction should be on the ones.

Decimals are an extension of the concept of place value and base 10. The place a digit holds in a number conveys its value, both for whole numbers and for decimal numbers. For example, in 147.9, the 9 is adjacent and to the right of the decimal point and to the right of the ones digit, 7. This is the place where digits have a base 10 value of tenths.

If there was another digit included on the decimal side of the decimal point, for example 147.96, then the 6 is in the one hundredths place. The 6 represents 6/100.

This is the case with money, for example with £16.45, the 4 represent 4 tenths (four 10 pence coins) of £1 and the 5 represents 5 hundredths (five 1 pence coins) of £1.

The place values can be seen in this example:

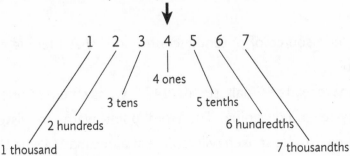

The centre of symmetry in place value is the ones

1 2 3 4 5 6 7

4 ones
3 tens
2 hundreds
1 thousand
5 tenths
6 hundredths
7 thousandths

Each consecutive 'place' is 10 times smaller in this direction.

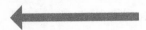

Each consecutive 'place' is 10 times bigger in this direction.

These rules apply across all the digits and that includes both sides of the decimal point.

One image that might be used to illustrate this place value concept is a metre rule. If one metre represents one, then ten centimetres (a decimetre) represent a tenth (1/10), one centimetre represents a hundredth (1/100) and one millimetre represents one thousandth (1/1000).

Another image could be created with the base 10 blocks. If the big cube represents 1 (instead of its normal role of representing 1000), then the 'flat square' represents one tenth (because 10 of them make 1), the 'long' block represents one hundredth and the small cube represents one thousandth.

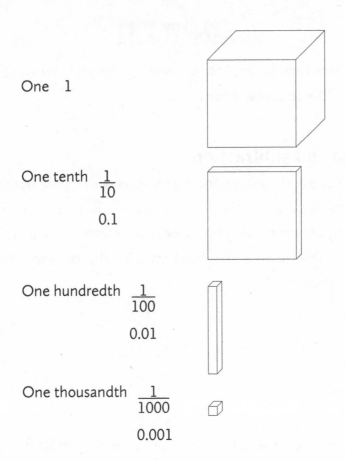

One   1

One tenth $\frac{1}{10}$

          0.1

One hundredth $\frac{1}{100}$

          0.01

One thousandth $\frac{1}{1000}$

          0.001

The relevance of the topic/concept to developing maths skills

Decimals are primarily about base 10 and about place value for quantities less than 1. They can be used to express any value less than 1. They can be linked to both fractions and percentages. They are involved in many aspects of everyday life, from money to measuring.

Decimal fractions are much easier to compare (for value) than fractions.

THE TASK

The task here is to be able to use decimal numbers when calculating with any of the four operations.

Addition and subtraction

The procedure and concept are the same as with whole numbers. The numbers to be added or the numbers to be subtracted must be lined up vertically according to place value. For example, to add 1.02 + 13.4 + 7.983 + 0.004 rewrite the numbers with the corresponding place values above each other:

$$
\begin{array}{r}
1.02 \\
13.4 \\
7.983 \\
+\,0.004 \\
\hline
\end{array}
$$

Note that the decimal points also line up (as they must if you line up place values).

The trading or renaming, if required, follows the same principle as with whole numbers, for example, 1 can be exchanged for 10 tenths, 1 tenth for 10 hundredths (and vice-versa).

Multiplication and division by decimal numbers

This requires the link between a decimal when written as 0.4 and as a fraction 4/10 to remind the student that the 4 in 0.4 is $4 \div 10$. The decimal disguises the $\div$ sign.

So, for multiplication by a decimal number that is less than 1, for example 52×0.4 is really two operations:

$52 \times 4 = 208$ and $208 \div 10 = 20.8$

And 52 × 0.04 is also two operations, one of them a division because 0.04 = 4/100 = 4 ÷ 100:

$$52 \times 4 = 208 \qquad \text{and} \qquad 208 \div 100 = 2.08$$

Dividing by a decimal number that is less than 1 also requires you to think about the concept of decimals.

For example, dividing by 5, 0.5 and 0.05, is dividing by 5, 5/10 and 5/100. The dividing number is 10 times smaller from 5 to 0.5 and 100 times smaller from 5 to 0.05.

When a number is divided by numbers that are progressively smaller, the answer gets progressively bigger. So, if the dividing number is 10 times smaller, the answer will be 10 times bigger, for example:

10 ÷ 5 = 2   (How many 5s in 10?)

  0.5 is 10× smaller than 5, so

10 ÷ 0.5 = 20   (How many halves in 10?)

  0.05 is 10× smaller than 0.5, so

10 ÷ 0.05 = 200   (How many five hundredths in 10?)

The answers to such divisions will be understood if the concepts of decimals and of division are understood.

Meta-cognition (thinking about how and what you are thinking)

To understand decimals, it is necessary to see them as an extension of the base 10 place value system.

It is easier to compare quantities expressed as decimals than when expressed as fractions. If the fractions that are difficult to compare are converted to decimals, then the comparison becomes much more straightforward. So, when dealing with quantities less than 1 it is useful to be able to draw on an interlinking knowledge of fractions, decimals and percentages and an understanding of that interlinking.

One way to check out a basic understanding of decimals is to count up in tenths...0.1, 0.2, 0.3, 0.4, 0.5, 0.6, 0.7, 0.8, 0.9...what comes next? It's *not* 0.10. That is not the required change in place value for the 1.

It sometimes helps to think of decimals as fractions, as tenths, hundredths, thousandths...1 tenth, 2 tenths, 3 tenths, 4 tenths, 5 tenths, 6 tenths, 7 tenths, 8 tenths, 9 tenths, 10 tenths. 10 tenths are 1. So, the tenths sequence ends with...0.8, 0.9, **1.0**. As with all counting in the base 10 system, when you reach 10 of whatever value you are counting, that takes you to the next place value.

Decimals can also be an experience that changes thinking about multiplication and division. If a number (whether bigger or smaller than 1) is *multiplied* by a decimal number that is less than 1, the answer will be smaller than the original number.

If some number (whether bigger or smaller than 1) is *divided* by a decimal number that is less than 1, the answer will be bigger than the original number.

The same rules apply when using fractions.

Things to do and practise

Practise counting on and back in decimals and do this across place values.

Round up decimals when shopping or looking at prices, for example, £1.95 to £2 and £399.99 to £400.

Add up the rounded prices on a shopping trip. Estimate the adjustment to make the addition accurate, for example, £2.95 + £7.99 is £3 + £8 = £11 when rounded up. The adjustment is 5p + 1p, so the accurate price is slightly lower than £11.00. It is £11.00 − 6p = £10.94.

Chapter 17

Multiplying and Dividing by 10, 100 and 1000 (Part 2)

The focus in Part 2 is on decimal numbers. The concept is still place value. The outcome of multiplication and division by 10 (and 100 and 1000 and any power of 10) remains the same as it did for whole numbers. Multiply by 10 and each digit in the number becomes 10 times bigger and moves up one place (value). Divide by 10 and each digit in the number becomes 10 times smaller ($\div$ 10) and moves down one place (value).

Multiplication

$0.5 \times 10 = 5$

The 5 in 0.5 is in the tenths place. It moves to the ones place when multiplied by 10.

$\dfrac{5}{10} \times 10 = 5$

$0.06 \times 10 = 0.6$

The 6 in 0.06 is in the hundredth place. It moves to the tenths place when multiplied by 10.

$\dfrac{6}{100} \times 10 = \dfrac{6}{10} = 0.6$

If 0.06 is multiplied by 100, the 6 will move from the hundredths place to the ones place:

$$0.06 \times 100 = 6$$

$$\frac{6}{100} \times 100 = 6$$

If the number being multiplied is more complex, for example 342.78 × 100 = 34278 focus on a digit. Here, the ones digit, 2, moves to the hundreds place and the other digits follow, maintaining the same sequence of digits. You could also focus on the hundredths digit, 8, which will move to the ones place.

The place value movement is to higher values, a move to the left. The decimal point is no longer needed in this example as there are no longer any digits representing decimal place values.

Division

$$5 \div 10 = 0.5$$

The 5 ones become 5 tenths when divided by 10, so the 5 moves from the ones place to the tenths place (value).

$$6 \div 100 = 0.06$$

The 6 ones become 6 hundredths when divided by 100, so the 6 moves from the ones place to the hundredths place (value).

$$34278 \div 100 = 342.78$$

The hundreds digit, 2, moves to the ones place and the other digits follow, maintaining the same sequence of digits. A decimal point is included to indicate the presence of digits that have a decimal value.

The place value movement is down to lower values, a move to the right.

Focus on a digit. Move it appropriately to the multiplication or division, for example 3 places bigger (to the left) for ×1000 or 3 places smaller (to the right) for ÷1000. Move the other digits, maintaining the same sequence of digits.

Chapter 18

Percentages

Percentages are probably the most user-friendly way of presenting numbers that are less than 1. They are also used for values greater than 1, as in the classic soccer coach quote, 'The lads gave it 110% today.' Percentages up to, but below, 100% are less than 1. A typical bank interest rate (2017) on savings is around 2%. A typical rate on a credit loan from a shop is 34%. (You don't need a degree in maths to see who gets the advantage there!)

I think of the symbol for percentages, % as having two zero symbols and thus it relates to 100, which also has two zero symbols.

The concept of percentages is, not surprisingly, a variation on the concepts of fractions and decimals.

1 is 100%.

For a half:

The fraction is ½ or 1 ÷ 2.

The decimal is 0.5 (which you get when you divide 1 by 2).

The percentage is 50%, which you get when you calculate: $\frac{1}{2} \times 100\%$.

A decimal can be converted to a percentage by multiplying by 100, for example, 0.27 × 100 = 27%.

A fraction can be converted to a decimal by dividing the top number by the bottom number, for example, for a half, this will be 1 ÷ 2 = 0.5.

A percentage can be converted to a decimal by dividing by 100, for example 47% ÷ 100 = 0.47.

An example of this relationship/sequence in action is a test mark of 17/20.

Fraction: $\dfrac{17}{20}$ Decimal: $17 \div 20 = 0.85$ Percentage: $0.85 \times 100 = 85\%$

A visual image of a 100 square can show the relative values of percentages up to 100. Of course, the image is also that used for a 1 to 100 square hence its familiarity and ease of use.

1	2	3	4	5	6	7	8	9	10
11	12	13	14	15	16	17	18	19	20
21	22	23	24	25	26	27	28	29	30
31	32	33	34	35	36	37	38	39	40
41	42	43	44	45	46	47	48	49	50
51	52	53	54	55	56	57	58	59	60
61	62	63	64	65	66	67	68	69	70
71	72	73	74	75	76	77	78	79	80
81	82	83	84	85	86	87	88	89	90
91	92	93	94	95	96	97	98	99	100

10%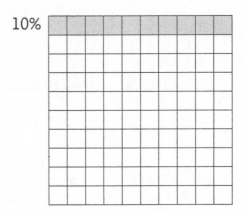

50% 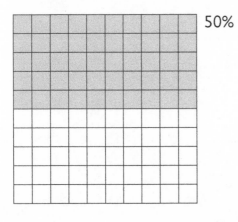 80%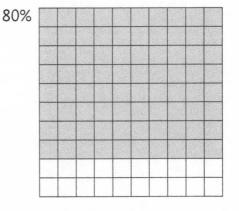

Key values for fractions, decimals and percentages

$\dfrac{1}{1}$ 1.0   100%

$\dfrac{1}{2}$ 0.5   50%

$\dfrac{1}{4}$ 0.25   25%

$\dfrac{1}{10}$ 0.1   10%

$\dfrac{1}{100}$ 0.01   1%

Key values can be used to access other values, for example:

$\dfrac{3}{4} = \dfrac{1}{2} + \dfrac{1}{4}$ 75% = 50% + 25%   0.75 = 0.5 + 0.25

20% = 2 × 10%   5% = ½ × 10%

Chapter 19

Word Problems

In a survey of teachers of special needs teachers in the USA (Bryant, Bryant and Hammill 2000), the researchers identified 33 tasks that were problematic for their students. The top three 'difficult' tasks were:

1. Has difficulty with word problems.

2. Has difficulty with multi-step problems.

3. Has difficulty with the language of math.

One of the reasons that students find maths problems difficult is that the problems often leave reality and common sense behind. For example:

'Bill baked 15 cupcakes in an hour. How many cupcakes could he bake in 4 hours?'

A student answered with, 'It depends how big his oven is.'

Students can be encouraged to make up word problems so that they learn for themselves the strategies that are used to make a problem less transparent than a computation.

They can also be shown the Singapore Model (Bar) Method (Kho Tek Hong *et al.* 2009) which uses a visual approach where quantities are represented by bars/rectangles, for example:

'85 boys and 97 girls went on a school trip. How many children went on the trip?'

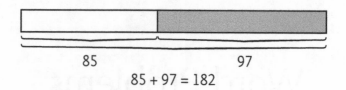

$$85 + 97 = 182$$

'A chef cooks 55 cakes. She has cooked 5 times as many cakes as she cooked bread rolls. How many bread rolls did she cook?'

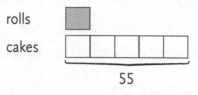

number of rolls × 5 = number of cakes = 55

number of rolls = 55 ÷ 5

A visual method for percentages

There are 400 pupils in a school. 40% are boys. How many are girls?

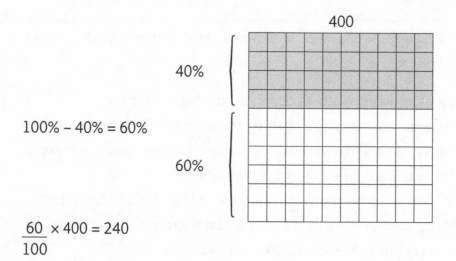

$$\frac{60}{100} \times 400 = 240$$

The visual images help to interpret the question rather than just relying on the words. This is an approach used throughout this book.

Chapter 20

Measurement

The metric units of measurement have a consistency. They are all based on 10 and powers of 10 and so relate to place value. Decimals are avoided, though not completely, using consistent prefixes.

Vocabulary and language

The prefixes used in measurement are useful information.

μ	micro	means one millionth	1/1 000 000
m	milli	means one thousandth	1/1000
c	centi	means one hundredth	1/100
k	kilo	means one thousand	1000
M	mega	means one million	1 000 000

The world of computers uses prefixes, including some for huge numbers, for example, a gigabyte is a billion bytes, 1 000 000 000 and a yottabyte is a million, million, million, million bytes or a billion, billion, million bytes, 1 000 000 000 000 000 000 000 000.

Once at a thousand, the prefixes are for multiples of 1000. For example, a thousand thousands, a million, is Mega and a thousand millions, a billion, is Giga.

Chapters 12 and 17 will be helpful when trying to convert within units, for example, kilometres to metres requires ×1000 and grams to kilograms requires ÷1000.

There is a need to be careful with place value when doing some conversions, for example:

To change 78 m to kilometres:

78 ÷ 1000 = 0.078km

A common error is 0.78 km. For this division, focus on the change in place value for the 8. In 78m it is 8 ones. When divided by 1000 it becomes 8 thousandths, 0.008. Then put in the 7 to give 0.078. Keep the sequence of digits.

Tens	Ones	.	Tenths	Hundredths	Thousandths	
7	8	.			8	Step 1
	0	.	0	7	8	Step 2

To change 2.93km to metres the most common error, caused by 'moving the decimal point three places' is 2093m. As there are only 2 digits after the decimal point, moving 3 places requires fitting in a zero. Without an understanding of the place values of the digits and with a purely mechanical 'move 3 places' some people insert a zero as shown. As ever, focus on a digit in 2.93. The 2 is 2 ones which will become 2 thousands, 2000. Now fit in the sequence of other digits to get 2930m.

Thousands	Hundreds	Tens	Ones	.	Tenths	Hundredths	
	8		2	.	9	3	
2							Step 1
2	9	3	0	.			Step 2

Chapter 21

Time

A clock is a circular number line with three sets of accompanying digits:

0–12   for hours   0–60   for minutes   0–60   for seconds

Time is such a challenging topic that it requires a book of its own (Chinn 2009), so this chapter is restricted to highlighting some of the problems that can occur and why that may be the case.

Time is another topic that challenges consistency. In fact, there are several challenges, maybe too many for young children to absorb. Another browse through the bookshelves of your local bookseller will reveal the age group at which books on time are targeted. It is probably too young. By trying to teach any topic too soon, there is a risk that the first learning experiences will be about failure, or be too confusing or presented before the pupil is ready, or all three.

Vocabulary and language

Time is full of problems with vocabulary and language, for example, 'quarter past 3' can generate a range of problems:

Quarter is a quarter of 60, which is 15. A common error, based on the experience of base 10 numbers is 25, a quarter of 100.

No units are mentioned. It is actually, '1 quarter of an hour past 3 hours'. *Past* means it is 3 hours *plus* a quarter of an hour.

'Quarter' comes before '3' yet the digital clock will show 3:15. (In the USA they say, 'A quarter after 3', which helps the order.)

And for a time such as 08:50 there are big problems interpreting it as it is sometimes said, '10 to 9'. That interpretation is a long way from literal. There would have to be a lot of prerequisite learning before that interpretation can be understood.

Images, symbols and concepts

Time is full of problems with images, symbols and concepts; for example, time uses base 12 and base 60 and a circular number line which represents different units (hours, minutes and seconds).

The relevance of the topic/concept to developing maths skills

It is not so much about the developmental benefits of learning time, but about its critical role in everyday life.

Meta-cognition (thinking about how and what you are thinking)

The learner must put aside much previous learning and interpret it in a new way.

Things to do and practise

Use a real clock, so that the hand movements are synchronised.

A digital clock or watch is only a partial answer. That will allow the learner to 'tell' the time, but not understand it, nor see relationships such as 2:15 being 45 minutes before 3 o'clock.

Chapter 22

Estimation

An Essential Maths Skill?

The first part of this chapter (until the 'Estimation and risk taking' heading) comes from an article which I wrote for the March 2012 edition of Special, the nasen magazine (Chinn 2012; reproduced with permission). I have included it because in many ways it summarises many of the themes within this short book.

There were four articles in the education press at the end of 2011 about maths that caught my interest. One was about the huge amount of money poured into 'Skills for Life' maths with little effect. The second was the Chief Inspector of Schools claiming that children 'have not learned their tables until they have instantaneous recall'. The third was from the Schools Minister who claimed that the use of calculators at a young age undermined arithmetical rigour. The fourth was that maths was the least popular subject for 15-year-old students.

The first and last articles suggest that there is something wrong with the way we are teaching maths. The second and third articles reveal beliefs from highly influential people about maths education that could be part of the problem with teaching this key subject.

I have claimed for many years now that much could be learned about teaching maths by looking at the children who struggle to learn maths. Many of these children will have special needs. Look to the 'outliers' for ideas for communicating maths to *all* learners.

I want to illustrate that claim by considering the skill of estimation and what factors are involved including student factors and maths factors. And I want to slip a few pragmatic thoughts into the mix.

We need our children, and thus our adults, to be engaged by maths, to have enough competence to deal, as a minimum goal, with 'the maths of life'. The two beliefs quoted at the start may contribute, alongside some other beliefs about maths, to the disengagement that begins for some children when they are very young.

I understand the importance of times table facts, but the need for instantaneous recall of every fact as acquired by rote, is harder for me to accept. This is not down to the maths. It is down to learners. Some children simply cannot achieve this goal, which brings me to *my* first belief. Persistent failure rarely motivates. Don't set goals that are unachievable for some children. Far too many children with special needs, and even those without, face a curriculum which generates too many experiences of failure. We need strong, but 'unanxious' expectations.

The fact that the money poured into the Skills for Life programme was ineffective and that maths is the least popular school subject for 15-year-olds suggest that there is something wrong, at a fundamental level, with the way maths is taught to too many of our students.

So, where does estimating come in?

Subitising

Brian Butterworth is the UK's top expert on dyscalculia. He believes that one of the key prerequisite skills for developing competence in maths is subitising, the ability to look at a small and random array of dots and know how many are there. This is, in effect, an early demonstration of a sense of number and quantity, a foundation on which maths ability can be built. I have taught 13-year-old severely dyslexic students who need to count my fingers when I show three and ask, 'How many?'

What I want to know about subitising is, how close do they get to the right answer when they are encouraged to guess, to estimate, or as my American colleague, a skilled estimator, once said, 'Controlled exploration'. I do not want to make this exercise a matter of 'right or wrong'. I want to invoke the wise words of one of my severely dyslexic American students, 'Close enough for government work'.

A lot of everyday maths is about being 'close enough for government work'. Students should be able to make their estimates in a low stress, low risk way thus developing their sense of number and discussing just how accurate they need to be according to the circumstances. This is leading to meta-cognition, thinking about how they are thinking, not just mindless 'doing maths and getting the right answer'.

Activities to develop this skill could include scattering coins or counters or looking at clusters of dots and estimating, 'How many?' Taking those random clusters and arranging objects in patterns can introduce bigger numbers, showing how to find the 'easy' numbers in the 'hard' numbers.

It can also be about reducing the number and length of times that children feel helpless. In maths 'not knowing' can often be addressed by using what you do know to work out, or maybe get close to what you need to know. Teachers need to sanction that approach. This can lead to children checking the reasonableness of answers, a process that is not done often enough. I am a fan of the question, when it is coupled with understanding, 'Is the "proper" answer bigger or smaller?'

Being numerically literal

Taking communications literally is not the exclusive preserve of children on the autism spectrum. In fact, I am sure that almost any characteristic you select from a special need will appear in some children without any identified 'difficulties'. I consider this trait to interpret numbers literally to be linked to the need for consistency and to thinking, or cognitive, style.

There is increasing support for introducing more meta-cognition into classrooms (and it has the benefit of being free). It would be discriminatory not to do this for children with special needs.

Back in the 1980s, along with some colleagues in the USA, I researched thinking style in mathematics (see Chapter 4). We identified the characteristics of two styles (see page 21). Most people use a mix of both styles, hopefully at the appropriate times. The 'grasshopper' thinker takes the big picture, overviews the problem, often estimates (effectively) and appraises answers. Grasshoppers have a good sense of number.

The 'inchworm' thinker relies on formulas, takes numbers literally, so that every fact stands alone creating a large load on memory, and is unlikely to check any answers.

Children who are heavily reliant on the inchworm approach are at risk in maths, especially if they have weak working and (mathematical) long-term memories, as is the case for many children with special needs. By not being able to link facts, concepts and procedures they can only rely on memory. So, for example, when learning the 121 basic addition facts, the task for them is 121 facts to learn. By taking a literal approach they fail to link facts such as 'doubles plus or minus 1' or the commutative facts. They do not link multiplication and addition or any of the basic concepts that make maths accessible and developmental. For them 9 is '9' and not 'one less than 10'.

There is a sense of consistency to be considered here, too. The security of $9 + 8$ being always 17 can be reassuring. But this fact can be rounded up and extended, for example, knowing that £90 + £80 = £170 and is almost £200 is a useful reality.

There are lots of games, exercises and discussions here that can be easily created to develop a better understanding of number and operation concepts. The guiding rules for creating these are both KISS, 'Keep it Simple (Stupid)' and the corresponding rule 'Keep it Successful (Stupid)'.

Calculators

Ministers of Education in the UK can be unequivocal at times, always a dangerous stance to take in any complex field. If they say that they don't approve of the use of calculators, then many teachers and other academics might feel like pointing out that it could be more complicated than that.

I was given my first calculator in 1965 when I was part way through my PhD (in applied physics). It was electrically powered, could only do the four operations and cost the same as my annual grant. It was also quite large. My PhD was not marked down because I used this machine.

The use of calculators cannot be viewed in isolation as being either good or bad. It depends on how they are used, of course, and how their use is linked to other educational factors, for example, thinking style or estimation skills.

So, a calculator should not be used if the child has no sense of number or ability to appraise the answer that the calculator shows. (Is that me being unequivocal?) The story is different for the combination of calculator plus estimation. And maybe the calculator could be part of the programme that develops a child's sense of number. If the keys are tapped correctly, in the correct order, then calculators give answers that are consistent and correct. More games and activities could be developed here!

Empty number lines (number lines without gradations)

'I work in dyslexia therefore I am multisensory.' This seemed to be a belief or even a mantra for quite a while. If we examine the implications of using apparatus and visual images, then it might be a very useful belief.

The empty number line is cheap and hugely effective as a visual aid when teaching estimation. A full number line encourages children to count, to stay at that fundamental level of number sense. An empty number line requires children to think of numbers as quantities and quantities that are inter-related. They can be used at different levels of skill, from 'Which is the bigger part?' to 'Estimate where 65 comes on this 0–100 number line' and later to fractions and proportion. Apparatus that encourages mathematical development has many advantages.

Mental arithmetic and estimation

To be successful at mental arithmetic you need a good working memory. Sadly, it is frequently the case that children with special needs have poor working memories. Add onto this the strange culture of maths where you are expected to answer mental arithmetic questions very quickly. That exacerbates the problem by increasing anxiety. It is, again, often the case that children with special needs tend to be slower at processing some information. Consequently, an accurate and fast performance at mental arithmetic tasks is unlikely.

Self-esteem is usually built on experiences of success. The same is true of motivation. Failure does not always spur children onwards, especially when they are not engrossed in a subject.

Differentiation can be achieved in the classroom by allowing answers to be estimates. And the bonus is that that ability is a life skill. When shopping or eating out I rarely check a bill by meticulously adding up all the items. I estimate. If I am worried by my estimate that there is an error, I might do an accurate addition. The same is true of percentages. I estimate and then discover that the offer on my credit card is somewhat biased towards the bank!

Estimation offers a pragmatic introduction to appraising answers. This brings us back to the evaluative question, 'Is the real answer going to be bigger or smaller than the estimate?'

Estimation and risk taking

The learning factors raised in this book are often interlinked. The maths topics, too, are often interlinked. For the inchworm learner, estimation, often perceived as 'guessing', is a risk. For the grasshopper learner, estimation is not guessing, it is controlled exploration. The extremely important issue of risk taking in maths can be addressed when teaching estimation. Children will avoid answering maths questions if they think they are going to be wrong. They simply don't try. This is that fear of negative evaluation. Estimation does not have that absolute judgement of right or wrong. Once children can be encouraged to risk a guess, an estimate, then the fear of being wrong is dramatically reduced.

Estimation and checking answers

When marking the 2000+ papers used to standardise my 15-minute maths screener test (Chinn 2017b) there were many occasions where the answer written down just could not be correct had it been appraised by even the wildest of estimates. As with the use of the calculator, evaluating an answer, and maybe even pre-estimating, is a great security blanket for the insecure mathematician.

Finally

Often a lesson is about 'What else are you teaching?' Not the main thrust of the lesson, but the bits, like revisiting prerequisites, like offering a new perspective on a concept, like building confidence and motivation with some positive and appropriate feedback. Estimation is a powerful tool for teaching many aspects of maths.

Is the answer bigger or smaller?

This question can be the first one used when estimating. For example, $456 \div 0.5$: 'Is the answer bigger or smaller than 456?' The division sign often means 'It's smaller' but here 'It's bigger.' It can be used for the appraisal of answers, for example, in the question from my standardised maths test, one answer given was

$$
\begin{array}{r}
103 \\
- 7 \\
\hline
104
\end{array}
$$

The answer cannot be bigger than 103.

A follow-up question that can be used is, 'Is the answer a lot bigger (or smaller)?'

These two questions can help build confidence and ability.

References and Further Reading

American Psychiatric Association (2013) *Diagnostic and Statistical Manual of Mental Disorders*. 5th edn. Arlington, VA: American Psychiatric Publishing.

Berch, D.B. (2005) 'Making sense of number sense: Implications for children with mathematical disabilities.' *Journal of Learning Disabilities 38*, 4, 333–339.

Bath, J.B., Chinn, S.J. and Knox, D.E. (1986) *The Test of Cognitive Style in Mathematics*. East Aurora, NY: Slosson.

Boaler, J. (2015) *The Elephant in the Classroom: Helping Children to Learn and Love Maths*. 2nd edn. London: Souvenir Press.

Bransford, J.D., Brown, A.L. and Cocking, R.R. (eds) (2000) *How People Learn*. Washington DC: National Academy Press.

Bryant, D.P., Bryant, B.R. and Hammill, D.D. (2000) 'Characteristic behaviours of students with LD who have teacher identified math weaknesses.' *Journal of Learning Disabilities 33*, 168–173.

Bugden, S. and Ansari, D. (2015) 'How Can Cognitive Developmental Neuroscience Constrain Our Understanding of Developmental Dyscalculia?' In S. Chinn (ed.) *The Routledge International Handbook of Dyscalculia and Mathematical Learning Difficulties*. London: Routledge.

Burden, R. (2005) *Dyslexia and Self-Concept*. London: Whurr.

Buswell, G.T. and Judd, C.M. (1925) Summary of educational investigations relating to arithmetic. *Supplementary Educational Monographs*. Chicago: University of Chicago Press.

Butterworth, B. (2003) *The Dyscalculia Screener*. London: GL Assessment.

Butterworth, B. and Yeo, D. (2003) *Dyscalcuia Guidance*. London: GL Assessment.

Chinn, S.J. (1995) 'A pilot study to compare aspects of arithmetic skill.' *Dyslexia Review 4*, 4–7.

Chinn, S.J. (2009) 'Mathematics anxiety in secondary school students in England.' *Dyslexia 15*, 61–68.

Chinn, S.J. (2012) 'The Power of Estimation.' *Special (nasen)*, March 2012, pp.14–16.

Chinn, S.J. (2013) 'Is the population really woefully bad at maths?' *Mathematics Teaching 232*, 25–28.

Chinn, S.J. (2017a) *The Trouble with Maths: A Practical Guide to Helping Learners with Numeracy Difficulties*. 3rd edn. Abingdon: Routledge.

Chinn, S.J. (2017b) *More Trouble with Maths: A Complete Guide to Identifying and Diagnosing Mathematical Difficulties*. 2nd edn. Abingdon: Routledge.

Chinn, S.J. and Ashcroft J.R. (1992) 'The Use of Patterns.' In T.R. Miles and E. Miles (eds) *Dyslexia and Mathematics*. London: Routledge.

Chinn, S.J. and Ashcroft, J.R. (2017) *Mathematics for Dyslexics and Dyscalculics: A Teaching Handbook*. 4th edn. Chichester: Wiley.

Chinn, S.J., McDonagh, D., Van Elswijk, R., Harmsen, H. *et al.* (2001) 'Classroom studies into cognitive style in mathematics for pupils with dyslexia in special education in the Netherlands, Ireland and the UK.' *British Journal of Special Education 28*, 2, 80–85.

Clausen-May, T. (2005) *Teaching Maths to Pupils with Different Learning Styles*. Two Thousand Oaks, CA: Paul Chapman Publishing.

DfES (2001) The National Numeracy Strategy. Guidance to Support Learners with Dyslexia and Dyscalculia. London. DfES. 0512/2001

Dowker, A. (2005) *Individual Differences in Arithmetic*. Hove/New York: Psychology Press.

Emerson, J. and Babtie, P. (2010) *The Dyscalculia Assessment*. London: Continuum.

Hattie, J. (2009) *Visible Learning*. London: Routledge.

Henderson, A. (2012) *Dyslexia, Dyscalculia and Mathematics. A Practical Guide*. Abingdon: Routledge.

Hornigold, J. (2015) *The Dyscalculia Pocket Book*. Alresford: Teachers' Pocketbooks.

Kavanagh, J.K. and Truss, J.T. (eds) (1988) *Learning Disabilities: Proceedings of the National Conference*. Parkton, MD: York Press.

Kho Tek Hong *et al.* (2009) *The Singapore Model Method*. Singapore: Ministry of Education.

Lane, C. and Chinn, S.J. (1986) 'Learning by self-voice echo.' *Academic Therapy 21*. 477–481.

Miles, T. and Miles, E. (eds) (2004) *Dyslexia and Mathematics*. 2nd edn. Abingdon/New York: Routledge.

Ofsted (2008) *Mathematics: Understanding the Score*. (Report on Primary and Secondary Mathematics). London: Ofsted. Accessed on 3 May 2018 at www.childrens-mathematics.net/continuity_ofsted_maths.pdf.

Orwell, G. (2000/1945) *Animal Farm*. London: Penguin.

Rashid, S. and Brooks, G. (2010) 'The levels of attainment in literacy and numeracy of 13 to 19-year-olds in England, 1948–2009.' *Literacy Today 32*, 1, 13–24.

Seligman, M. (1998) *Learned Optimism*. New York: Pocket Books.

Skemp, R.R. (1986) *The Psychology of Learning Mathematics*. London: Penguin.

Usiskin, Z. (1998) 'Paper and Pencil Algorithms in a Calculator and Computer Age.' In L. Morrow and M. Kennedy (eds) *The Teaching and Learning of Algorithms in School Mathematics*. Reston, VA: NCTM.

Yeo, D. (2003) *Dyslexia, Dyspraxia and Mathematics*. London: Whurr.

Publications by Steve Chinn

2009   *What to Do When You Can't Tell the Time.* Egon. *(Does what it says in the title.)*

2010   *Addressing the Unproductive Behaviours of Students with Special Needs.* Jessica Kingsley Publishers. *(Nominated for a nasen award.)*

2017   *Mathematics for Dyslexics and Dyscalculics: A Teaching Handbook.* 4th edn (with J.R. Ashcroft). Wiley. *(For a comprehensive coverage of theory and practice. A seminal text.)*

2017a   *The Trouble with Maths: A Practical Guide to Helping Learners with Numeracy Difficulties.* 3rd edn. David Fulton/Routledge. *(For a pragmatic approach to teaching and learning maths. The 1st edition won a nasen/TES book award in 2004.)*

2017b   *More Trouble with Maths: A Complete Guide to Identifying and Diagnosing Mathematical Difficulties.* 2nd edn. David Fulton/Routledge/nasen. *(For standardised tests and a range of other tests and clinical activities to use to create a comprehensive assessment/diagnosis.)*

2017   *Numicon Big Ideas* (with Fiona Goddard and Liz Henning). OUP. *(For a collection of lesson plans and supporting materials addressing the key ideas in maths for children who failed to grasp them securely first time.)*

2015   *The Routledge International Handbook of Dyscalculia and Mathematical Learning Difficulties.* (edited by Steve Chinn) Routledge. *(For a comprehensive overview from authors around the world covering classroom to neuroscience.)*

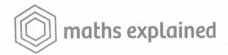

Low-cost video tutorials by Steve Chinn, extending the approach and ideas in this book, are available from www.mathsexplained.co.uk.

Index